Orofacial Pain

Oxford University Press makes no representation, express or implied, that the drug dosages in this book are correct. Readers must therefore always check the product information and clinical procedures with the most up-to-date published product information and data sheets provided by the manufacturers and the most recent codes of conduct and safety regulations. The authors and the publishers do not accept responsibility or legal liability for any errors in the text or for the misuse or misapplication of material in this work.

▶ Except where otherwise stated, drug doses and recommendations are for the non-pregnant adult who is not breast-feeding.

Orofacial Pain

Edited by

Joanna M. Zakrzewska

Consultant and Hon Professor,
Lead Clinician for Facial Pain,
Eastman Dental Hospital,
University College London Hospitals NHS Foundation Trust,
London, UK

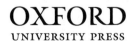

OXFORD
UNIVERSITY PRESS

OXFORD
UNIVERSITY PRESS

Great Clarendon Street, Oxford OX2 6DP

Oxford University Press is a department of the University of Oxford.
It furthers the University's objective of excellence in research, scholarship,
and education by publishing worldwide in

Oxford New York

Auckland Cape Town Dar es Salaam Hong Kong Karachi
Kuala Lumpur Madrid Melbourne Mexico City Nairobi
New Delhi Shanghai Taipei Toronto

With offices in

Argentina Austria Brazil Chile Czech Republic France Greece
Guatemala Hungary Italy Japan South Korea Poland Portugal
Singapore Switzerland Thailand Turkey Ukraine Vietnam

Oxford is a registered trade mark of Oxford University Press
in the UK and in certain other countries

Published in the United States
by Oxford University Press Inc., New York

British Library Cataloguing in Publication Data

Data available

Library of Congress Cataloging in Publication Data

Data available

Typeset by Newgen Imaging Systems (P) Ltd., Chennai, India
Printed in Great Britain
on acid-free paper by
Clays Ltd, St Ives plc

ISBN 978–0–19–923669–5

10 9 8 7 6 5 4 3 2 1

Contents

Preface

Welcome to our small book on orofacial pain which is addressed to all healthcare practitioners–dental, medical, or allied, under-graduate or postgraduate–who see patients with facial pain.

Recent epidemiological studies on the prevalence of orofacial pain in the community in the UK identified that 7% of the population had chronic orofacial pain and just under 50% sought healthcare advice. Patients consult doctors and dentists who often have radically different approaches which results in varying treatments. Patients, thus, often become confused and feel abandoned as they move between different healthcare professionals trying to find a cure.

Management of orofacial pain has improved dramatically over the years and it is now essential that everyone is aware of these advances so that our approach to the patient with facial pain is more consistent. To ensure that this book achieves this aim I chose an international multi-disciplinary panel of authors.

Orofacial pain experts from round the world acted as knowledge managers – finding, filtering and then critically appraising the literature. They then worked in teams of two or three in order to interpret this material in the light of their considerable clinical expertise. I chose clinical specialists from a range of different backgrounds to ensure that we achieved as wide a perspective as possible, so the authors include dentists with a special interest in facial pain, an epidemiologist, a neurologist, a neurosurgeon, an oral radiologist, oral surgeons, oral physiologists, oral physicians, psychologist, and a psychiatrist.

Having taken this evidence based psychosocial approach to the diagnosis and management of these patients we have presented the results using a mixture of mind maps, tables and short texts to ensure that you can access the material quickly in a clinical setting. A few key references should enable you to find the appropriate in-depth references and internet sites which may also be of use to your patients. The first five chapters are general and apply to all patients with pain or more specifically facial pain. Chapters 6 to 12 deal with specific types of facial pain and in Chapter 13 we speculate on how our diagnosis and management may change as a result of our growing knowledge of genetics. This book is a companion book to other larger works on this topic and also to the rest of the series.

We hope that this clinical manual will enable you to manage facial pain patients in a holistic empathic way and that you will encourage them to self manage by providing them with information. Patients need to feel believed, to know that all attempts have been made to come to a diagnosis and that appropriate treatment or referral has been carried out.

I am very grateful to all my authors for giving up some of their busy time to share in putting this book together and for working so well as a team. There will no doubt be omissions or over emphasis in certain areas and I take full responsibility for these as I heavily edited the book.

Thank you, for taking the time to read this.

To cure sometimes, to relieve often and to comfort always.

Joanna Zakrzewska

Contributors

Lene Baad-Hansen, DDS, PhD

Assistant Professor
Department of Clinical Oral Physiology
School of Dentistry,
University of Aarhus,
Denmark

Raymond A. Dionne, DDS, PhD

Scientific Director
National Institute of Nursing Research
National Institutes of Health Bethesda
Maryland, USA

Mark Drangsholt, DDS, PhD

Assistant Professor
Departments of Oral Medicine
and Dental Public Health Sciences
University of Washington
Seattle, WA, USA

**Charlotte Feinmann, MD,
MRCPsych, MSc**

Reader Liaison Psychiatry
University College London, UK

Heli Forssell, DDS, Odont. Dr

Chief Specialist
Department of Oral Diseases
and Pain Clinic
Turku University Hospital
Turku, Finland

Steven Graff Radford, DDS

Director
The Program for Headache and Orofacial
Pain, The Pain Center, Cedars-Sinai
Medical Center,
Adjunct Professor
UCLA School of Dentistry
Clinical Professor,
USC School of Dentistry
Los Angeles, CA, USA

**Miriam Grushka, MSc, DDS,
PhD**

Active Staff
William Osler Health Centre
Etobicoke Campus,
Department of Surgery and Private
Practice, Toronto, Canada

**Suthipun Jitpimolmard,
MD, DCN, FRCP**

Professor of Neurology
Department of Medicine
Faculty of Medicine
Director of Research and
Development Institute
Khon Kaen University, Thailand

Linda LeResche, ScD

Professor
Department of Oral Medicine
University of Washington
Seattle, WA, USA

Mark E. Linskey, M.D.

Associate Professor and
Chairman, Department of
Neurological Surgery
University of California
Irvine,
CA, USA

**Thomas List, DDS,
Odont. Dr.**

Professor, Orofacial Pain Unit
Dept. of Stomatognathic Physiology
Faculty of Odontology
Malmö University
Malmö,
Sweden

CONTRIBUTORS

Toby Newton-John, PhD, MPsych
Clinical Psychologist and Program
Director, Innervate Pain Management,
Newcastle Australia; and Faculty
of Medicine, University of Sydney
Australia

**Suk Ng, PhD, BDS, BSc,
FDSRCS Eng, DDRRCR**
Senior Lecturer/Honorary Consultant
Programme Director of Distance Learning
MSc in Dental and Maxillofacial Radiology
Department of Dental Radiology
King's College London Dental Institute at
Guy's, King's College
and St Thomas' Hospitals
London, UK

Richard Ohrbach, DDS, PhD
Associate Professor
Department of Oral Diagnostic Sciences
University at Buffalo
Buffalo, New York, USA

x

Jeffrey P Okeson, DMD
Professor and Chair, Department of Oral
Health Science
Director, Orofacial Pain Program
University of Kentucky College
of Dentistry
Lexington, Kentucky, USA

**Christian S. Stohler, D.M.D.,
Dr.Med.Dent.**
Professor and Dean
University of Maryland, Dental School
Baltimore, Maryland, USA

**Peter Svensson, DDS, PhD,
Dr.Odont.**
Professor and Chair, Department of
Clinical Oral Physiology School of
Dentistry, University of Aarhus
Clinical Consultant, Department of
Oral and Maxillofacial Surgery
Aarhus University Hospital
Denmark

**E. Russell Vickers,
MDS, PhD**
Dept of Anaesthesia and Pain
Management
University of Sydney
Sydney, Australia

Alain Woda, PhD
Professor
Faculty of Dentistry
Université d'Auvergne
Clermont-Ferrand, France

**Joanna M. Zakrzewska, MD,
FDSRCS, FFDRCSI**
Consultant and Hon Professor,
Lead Clinician for Facial Pain
Eastman Dental Hospital
University College London Hospitals
NHS Foundation Trust
London, UK

Abbreviations

AAN	American Academy of Neurology
ACE	Angiotensin converting enzyme
AED	Antiepileptic drugs
AFP	Atypical facial pain
AO	Atypical odontalgia
AV	Arterio-venous
BMS	Burning mouth syndrome
CNS	Central nervous system
CT	Computed tomography
DASS	Depression Anxiety Stress Scale
EFNS	European Federation of Neurological Societies
EMG	Electromyography
ESR	Erythrocyte sedimentation rate
FDA	US Food and Drug Administration
GCA	Giant cell arteritis
GPN	Glossopharyngeal neuralgia
IASP	International Association for the Study of Pain
ICRP	International Commission on Radiological Protection
IHS	International Headache Society
MPQ	McGill Pain Questionnaire
MRI	Magnetic resonance imaging
NSAID	Non-steroidal anti-inflammatory drugs
PET	Positron emission tomography
PHN	Post herpetic neuralgia
PIFP	Persistent idiopathic facial pain
QST	Quantitative sensory testing
RCT	Randomized, controlled trials
RDC/TMD	Research Diagnostic Criteria for Temporomandibular Disorders
SNRI	Serotonin noradrenaline re-uptake inhibitors
SSRI	Serotonin re-uptake inhibitors
SUNCT	Short lasting unilateral neuralgiform headache attacks with conjunctival injection and tearing

TAC	Trigeminal autonomic cephalalgias
TENS	Transcutaneous electrical nerve stimulation
TMD	Temporomandibular disorder
TMJs	Temporomandibular joints
TN	Trigeminal neuralgia

Chapter 1

Epidemiology of orofacial pain

Mark Drangsholt and Linda LeResche

> **Key points**
> - Definitions of epidemiological terms provided
> - Epidemiologic data can help in diagnosis, prediction of risk factors, prognosis and effect of treatment outcomes
> - The most common orofacial pain conditions include pulpitis, TMD, chronic idiopathic facial pains, and headaches
> - Orofacial pain has a considerable impact on quality of life.

1.1 Chapter plan

Figure 1.1 is an outline of the main contents of the chapter.

1.2 Definitions

1.2.1 What is epidemiology?

Epidemiology is the study of the distribution, determinants and natural history of disease in populations. Epidemiology first focused on well-defined disorders, such as infectious diseases, and now has been successfully applied to common chronic conditions such as cancer or heart disease. More recently, epidemiologic methods are used to study symptoms such as pain and other problems for which the definition of who is a case is based on self-report, or a combination of self report and clinical findings.

Figure 1.1 Plan of chapter

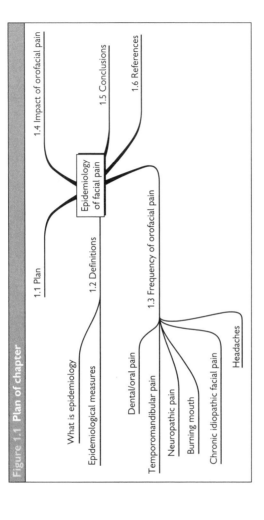

1.1 Plan

What is epidemiology

Epidemiological measures

1.2 Definitions

Epidemiology of facial pain

1.4 Impact of orofacial pain

1.5 Conclusions

1.6 References

1.3 Frequency of orofacial pain

Dental/oral pain

Temporomandibular pain

Neuropathic pain

Burning mouth

Chronic idiopathic facial pain

Headaches

Epidemiology can aid the pain clinician in a number of ways:

- knowing how common disorders are in the population, as well as their rates in specific age and sex groups, can aid the clinician in determining the most probable diagnosis in a particular case. For example, if a 21-year-old woman reports severe pain in the cheek region, the odds are much greater that she is suffering from a temporomandibular disorder (TMD) than from trigeminal neuralgia. In addition, the setting in which care is delivered is important in estimating the probability of diagnoses, since patients are less likely to present with rare or uncommon diagnoses in general practice or the community than in specialty, hospital or teaching institutions.

- factors associated with developing or having the disorder, or risk factors, can help to identify which people are more probable to have a diagnosis than others, or can help to identify causative factors.

- studies which follow people over time, or longitudinal studies, can help to define which subjects have a better clinical course or prognosis than others.

- studies, preferably with controls, and ultimately with random assignment (called randomized controlled trials) can be performed to definitively decide which therapies are more effective and which are less effective for specific pain conditions.

Figure 1.2 summarizes the use of epidemiology for the clinician.

1.2.2 **Basic epidemiologic measures**

Prevalence is the proportion of the population with a condition at a given point in time. Incidence is the rate of onset of new cases of a condition over a specific time period, usually a year.

Incidence and prevalence are related such that:

$$Prevalence = Incidence \times Mean\ Duration.$$

The number of cases in the population at any given time is a function of not only the rate at which new cases occur, but also how long the condition typically lasts. If the rate of onset of two conditions is the same, but one lasts one year and the other lasts two years, twice as many cases of the second condition will be found at any given time. Although pain arising from caries and periodontal disease is generally acute especially if treatment is provided, most other orofacial pain conditions in the population follow a chronic-recurrent course. Most of the epidemiologic data we have on orofacial pain are prevalence data.

In the epidemiologic sense, risk is defined as the likelihood that people without a disease, but who are exposed to certain factors (called risk factors) will acquire the disease. It is useful to think about two kinds of risk factors: those that we can do something about—like smoking—known as 'modifiable' risk factors; and those that we cannot – like age and sex – sometimes called 'risk indicators.'

Figure 1.2 Uses of epidemiology for clinicians

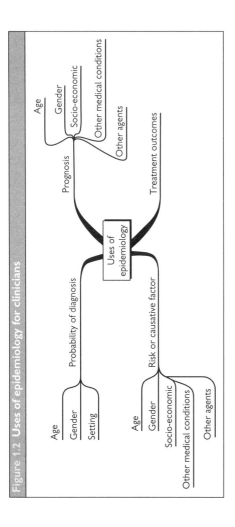

1.3 **Frequency of orofacial pain in the community**

Although a number of studies have investigated orofacial pain in specialty clinics, and some studies have looked at rates of specific types of pain (e.g. TMD) in the community, few have looked at all types of orofacial pain in people in the community, and not necessarily presenting for care in an office or clinic. Two studies, performed in the UK, asked about 2500 adult people in a postal questionnaire, whether they had '...had any pain in the face, mouth or jaws that lasted for one day or longer in the past month?' The range of 'yes' responses ranged from 12 to 19%, and most of these people were further examined by experts to provide a final diagnosis. These data provide some of the only population-based information on the frequency of various orofacial pain conditions. A compilation of the approximate percentage of the most common disorders, split into three groups, dentoalveolar, musculoligamentous/ soft tissue, and neurological/vascular, is listed in Table 1.1. Disorders that occurred less than 0.1% of the time are not listed. Please note that only the primary diagnosis is listed; the majority of orofacial pain patients will have more than one pain diagnosis at any given time, i.e. chronic idiopathic facial pain plus a temporomandibular disorder.

5

Table 1.1 Prevalence of face, mouth or jaw pain in the community		
Rank	Condition	1 month prevalence
Dento-alveolar		
1	irreversible/chronic pulpitis	1.2%
2	dental abscess	0.7%
3	sinusitis	0.7%
4	periodontal disease	0.5%
5	pericoronitis	0.4%
6	reversible pulpitis/dentin sensitivity	0.3%
Musculoligamentous/ soft tissue		
1	TMD pains – all types	1.5%
2	chronic tension-type headache	0.8%
3	recurrent oral ulcers	0.4%
4	lichen planus	0.1%
5	sore throat	0.1%
Neurological/vascular		
1	chronic idiopathic facial pain*	0.9%
2	migraine headache – all types	0.6%
3	neuropathic pain/nerve damage	0.2%
4	trigeminal neuralgia – all types	0.3%

* Also known as atypical odontalgia, atypical facial pain. Combined and adapted from MacFarlane, 2004 and Aggarwal, 2007.

Toothache, or irreversible pulpitis, is the most common diagnosis among the dento-alveolar group, TMD pain in the musculoligamentous, and chronic idiopathic orofacial pain (also known as atypical odontalgia/atypical facial pain) in the neurological/vascular category. It should be noted that people with headaches commonly report pains in the face or jaws, which explains the presence of these conditions in the table. In addition, these percentages may seem lower than other published reports, but the time period is for only one month, decreasing the number of people with the condition compared to the more commonly used 3, 6 or 12 month time periods.

1.3.1 **Toothache, periodontal and oral soft tissue pain**

Because caries is the most common cause of pain in the teeth, the prevalence of toothache in a population depends on the rate of caries and the factors that influence that rate – for example, diet, social class and levels of fluoride in the water supply (Chapter 6).

One US national study found an overall prevalence of toothache in the past 6 months among adults of 12%, with little difference in prevalence rates for men and women. Rates decreased with age from 17% in 18–34 year olds to 3% among those 75 or older. Toothache is likely the most common cause of orofacial pain among children. In one study of Australian school children, about 12% were found to have experienced at least one toothache before their fifth birthday, and almost one third (32%) had experienced toothache by the age of 12 years.

Few epidemiologic investigations of pain in the periodontal and oral soft tissues have been conducted. Population-based studies of herpes simplex and aphthous stomatitis, common oral lesions that typically cause acute, self-limiting pain, have found point prevalences around 1–2%. Pericoronitis, an acute infection around erupting third molars, commonly causes acute pain and trismus among persons in their late teens or early 20's.

1.3.2 **Temporomandibular Disorder (TMD) pain**

Temporomandibular disorders are musculoskeletal conditions characterized by pain in the temporomandibular joint and/or the associated muscles of mastication (Chapter 9). TMD pain is by far the most common of the chronic orofacial pain conditions, and it is similar to back pain in its intensity, persistence, and psychological impact. TMD pain is rare in children prior to puberty. Rates range from 9%–15% for women and from 3%–10% for men. Interestingly, TMD pain appears to be 1.5–2 times more common in women than in men in nearly every study. Also, in all studies where there was a clear pattern for age-specific prevalence, the peak age was around 35–45 years.

The few studies of onset rates of TMD pain that have been conducted, indicate that incidence rates of TMD pain are on the order of 2%–3% per year. This fairly low incidence of TMD suggests that the high prevalence of TMD pain in the population is due to its relatively long duration, rather than high rates of onset.

Recent epidemiologic research has investigated risk factors for TMD pain and these are discussed in Chapter 9 and Figure 9.2.

1.3.3 **Neuropathic, neurological pain and neuralgias**

Neuropathic pain is initiated or caused by a lesion in the nervous system so the pain is reported as being along the distribution of a nerve. With the high density of multiple cranial and other nerves in the face, mouth and head region, it is not surprising that an increasing number of orofacial pain conditions are thought to belong in this category.

Epidemiologic studies, like clinical experience, support the observation that risk of acquiring trigeminal neuralgia (TN) (Chapter 10) increases with age, and is more common in women. Other risk factors possibly associated with TN are multiple sclerosis, hypertension, and abstinence from alcohol and tobacco.

1.3.3.1 *Burning mouth pain (oral dysesthesia)*

There are few population-based studies of dysesthesias characterized by burning pain or discomfort in the oral soft tissues (Chapter 7). In a large study of US households, less than 1% of the population reported 'a prolonged unexplained burning sensation in your tongue or any other part of your mouth.' Rates were somewhat higher in women than in men. The rate of burning mouth pain increases with age, especially in the very elderly. Being female also seems to increase the risk of burning mouth pain. Some have speculated that loss of hormones with menopause may increase the risk of these conditions, but the research on this subject is far from clear.

1.3.3.2 *Chronic idiopathic facial pain (atypical odontalgia and atypical facial pain)*

Two conditions of great interest to clinicians are atypical odontalgia, which is localized, usually throbbing pain in a tooth or tooth site without identifiable pathology, and chronic idiopathic facial pain (atypical facial pain) — continuous, nagging, deep, diffuse pain in the absence of other pain diagnoses and identifiable pathology (Chapter 8). There is increasing evidence that a majority of these conditions are neuropathic in mechanism, although this is presently uncertain. Unfortunately, no population-based data exist on either of these conditions. One survey of 256 female patients of a single endodontist indicated that about 3% still had persistent tooth pain at least one month after endodontic treatment was completed. A longitudinal study of 175 persons with either initial or repeated root canal therapy reported that 12% had pain after at least one year, even though clinical and radiographic exams were normal. However, some of these subjects may have had persistent pain at the start of the study, explaining the high prevalence.

Clinical studies indicate that women are much more likely than men to seek care for chronic idiopathic facial pain and that the mean age of persons seeking care is around 40–55 years. The longitudinal study of root canal patients just cited showed that being female, having previous chronic pain conditions, or reporting pre-existing tooth pain were strong risk factors for persistent pain after a year or more. High rates of psychological disturbance also seem to occur in clinic populations of persons with chronic idiopathic facial pain but again, it is unclear whether these disturbances precede or follow the unremitting pain, and whether these differences are associated with having the pain problem, or with seeking care.

1.3.3.3 *Headaches*

Headache pain can commonly cross the artificial boundaries that medical and dental clinicians have created when dealing with head and neck pain. There is a large epidemiologic literature on headaches and on migraine headache in particular (Chapter 11). Migraine is more prevalent in women than in men, and prevalence varies with age, peaking between age 35 and 45 for both genders. At this age, prevalence averages about 7% for men and 20% for women. Non-migrainous headaches (primarily tension-type headaches) are extremely common conditions experienced by 60%–80% of adults. The prevalence on non-migrainous headache is higher in women than in men, but the gender difference is smaller than for migraine.

1.4 **The impact of orofacial pain**

Pain can disrupt a number of aspects of everyday life, including work, social and recreational activities, and sleep. A study of residents of Toronto found the most common impact of orofacial pain was worrying about one's health, which was experienced by over 70% of persons reporting pain. Forty-four percent of those with pain consulted a doctor or dentist; about 29% took medication; 14% reported sleep disturbance; and 4%–8% reported taking time off from work, staying in bed or avoiding their family and friends. The more severe the pain, the more likely people were to report significant impacts. While TMD is less likely than back pain or headache to interfere with work activity, many persons with TMD experience substantial psychological impact and disruption of social and recreational activities.

1.5 **Conclusion**

Good epidemiologic data on orofacial pain are not always currently available. For example, among the acute pain conditions, we know a great deal about the prevalence and distribution of toothache, but little about the prevalence of periodontal pain. There are some population-based data for burning mouth and trigeminal neuralgia but no population-based data are available for the unusual and difficult-to-treat conditions of chronic idiopathic facial pain and its possible variant atypical odontalgia. Well-conducted epidemiologic studies of these conditions could yield information highly relevant to their etiology, diagnosis, treatment and prognosis.

Aggarwal, V.R., McBeth, J., Lunt, M., Zakrzewska, J.M., Macfarlane, G.J. (2007). Development and validation of classification criteria for idiopathic orofacial pain for use in population-based studies. *Journal of Orofacial Pain,* **21**: 203–15.

Drangsholt, M., LeResche, L. (1999). Temporomandibular disorder pain. In (eds) Crombie I.K., Croft P.R., Linton S.J., LeResche L., Von Korff M., *Epidemiology of Pain.* pp. 203–33. IASP Press, Seattle.

LeResche, L., Mancl, L.A., Drangsholt, M., Huang, G., Von Korff, M. (2007). Predictors of onset of facial pain and temporomandibular disorders in early adolescence. *Pain,* **129**: 269–78.

Lipton, J.A., Ship, J.A., Larach-Robinson, D. (1993). Estimated prevalence and distribution of reported orofacial pain in the United States. *Journal American Dental Association,* **124**: 115–21.

Locker, D., Grushka, M. (1987). The impact of dental and facial pain. *Journal Dental Research,* **66**: 1414–17.

Macfarlane, T.V., Blinkhorn, A.S., Craven, R., Zakrzewska, J.M., Atkin, P., Escudier, M.P., Rooney, C.A., Aggarwal, V., Macfarlane, G.J. (2004). Can one predict the likely specific orofacial pain syndrome from a self-completed questionnaire? *Pain,* **111**: 270–7.

Scher, A.I., Stewart, W.F., Lipton, R.B. (1999). Migraine and headache: A meta-analytic approach. In (eds) Crombie, I,K., Croft, P.R., Linton, S.J., LeResche L., Von Korff, M. (eds.) *Epidemiology of Pain.* pp. 159–70 Seattle: IASP Press.

Chapter 2

History and examination

Russell Vickers and Joanna M. Zakrzewska

Key points

- Pain is common and invisible – a comprehensive history is mandatory
- Chronic pain is a complex biopsychosocial phenomenon
- Good communication skills improve the value of the history
- Multiple pain states and regions can be related
- Psychosocial history and comorbid anxiety/depression is important
- Clinical examination needs to exclude infection and occult pathology.

2.1 Chapter plan

Figure 2.1 is an outline of the main contents of this chapter.

2.2 Importance of history

A good history enables:

- Diagnosis to be made
- Severity of symptoms to be gauged and their effect
- Prognosis determined
- Tailoring of investigations
- Interpretation of results more accurately
- Placing of the patients' condition within the context of their social and psychological circumstances.

Taking a history is an interview not an investigation and this can be improved by adhering to this strategy as suggested by Bird and Cohen-Cole.

Presentation: create the right environment, introduce yourself with a handshake, and make the patient feel comfortable both physically and psychologically. Ensure that the patient knows that you will safeguard their confidentiality, give them the impression that you have plenty of time or tell them

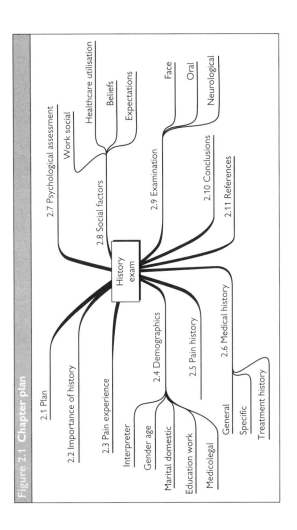

Figure 2.1 Chapter plan

History exam

- 2.1 Plan
- 2.2 Importance of history
- 2.3 Pain experience
- 2.4 Demographics
  - Interpreter
  - Gender age
  - Marital domestic
  - Education work
  - Medicolegal
- 2.5 Pain history
- 2.6 Medical history
  - General
  - Specific
  - Treatment history
- 2.7 Psychological assessment
- 2.8 Social factors
  - Work social
  - Healthcare utilisation
  - Beliefs
  - Expectations
- 2.9 Examination
  - Face
  - Oral
  - Neurological
- 2.10 Conclusions
- 2.11 References

up front how much time you have, prevent interruptions and explain the role/purpose of the meeting.

Empathy: patients need to feel that you understand them and that you too have emotions.

- Respect your patients' behaviour
- Support patients emotions, feelings
- Organize your time and agenda.

Be non-judgmental: you need to accept the person, not necessarily the behaviour, remain neutral.

Alliance and partnership: you need to ensure that it occurs on an equal basis.

Leave taking: ensure that you make it clear that there is a commitment on both sides to further management.

2.3 **Pain experience**

The stages of pain experience involve the following areas:

- *Nociception* – the physiological events that are transmitting the information to the brain
- *Perception* – the physical, spatial and temporal qualities of the pain
- *Appraisal* – the beliefs and expectations, how the current pain fits in with the past memory of pain
- *Behaviour* – the activities that contribute to the pain, the activities that result from the pain, e.g. non verbal behaviour, eating.

Complex pain states must therefore be deconstructed, with the separate components of the pain being measured and treated. Each patient has his/her 'pain story' that must be told to the clinician so that they 'understand my pain'. It therefore takes time to really understand months or years of pain, suffering and distress and so the British Pain Society suggests that a 45-minute consultation is necessary. Pain is an invisible symptom with multiple interrelated effects. A comprehensive written biopsychosocial assessment (patient completed pain questionnaire) allows the clinician to focus on the important aspects of the patient's history. This is necessary to identify biological disease states and psychological morbidity in order to ensure a correct clinical (multiaxial) diagnosis. Questionnaires that are of use will be discussed in Chapter 3.

2.4 **Demographics**

2.4.1 **Is an interpreter or chaperone needed?**

Qualified interpreters help the clinician to understand cultural differences in the meaning of pain and ensure a lack of bias. A chaperone (or partner) can correct a long complex pain history when the patient is a poor pain historian but may add their own interpretation to the history. Table 2.1 provides some hints on working with an interpreter.

2.4.2 Sex and age

There is a greater prevalence of older females with chronic orofacial pain, e.g. neuropathic pain, trigeminal neuralgia, temporomandibular disorder (TMD) and burning mouth syndrome. It is also known that more females seek healthcare and so predominate in the specialist centres.

2.4.3 Marital and domestic status

Does the patient's partner (or another family member) offer the necessary psychological and financial support, or is s/he a potential trigger or causal factor of emotional stress and suffering? There is the patient's 'pain' and the larger 'pain problem' that may involve other people in decreasing or increasing pain through background stress. Are there any other family members with chronic pain? It may be difficult to improve one person's pain due to complex psychosocial conditioning where other family members have chronic pain.

2.4.4 Education and current work

Low levels of education and unemployment correlate to increased pain prevalence and intensity. Will the patient understand the need for psychological assessment or will s/he view this as an intrusion? Will the patient be competent in order to comply with multiple treatments and polypharmacy?

2.4.5 Medico-legal issues

Is the pain related to a legal or insurance claim? Delays in the legal system can cause frustration and anger increasing pain intensity. Alternatively if there is the possibility of secondary financial gain from a 'pain and suffering' claim then it may be pragmatic for the patient to forcibly negate any improvement from pain treatments.

Table 2.1 Working with an interpreter

- Check that interpreter and patient speak same language/dialect
- Check that the interpreter is acceptable to the patient and trusted – may need to be same gender
- Discuss before the consultation the content of the interview and how you want to work
- Encourage the interpreter to interject if necessary
- Use easy language
- Observe interpreter and patient to pick up non verbal behaviours – may not be possible if done through a language telephone line
- Check that patient has understood by asking for feedback
- Leave yourself extra time
- Ensure patient has time to raise questions
- After the consultation check with interpreter how the interview went.

2.5 **Pain history**

Figure 2.2 lists the essential components of any pain history and all of the conditions described in the book will use this format.

2.5.1 **Describe your pain?**

Allow the patient to 'tell their story'. An accurate description from a patient can provide valuable information as to the diagnosis. For example:

- 'Excruciating pain in my teeth and face when I touch it or go out in the cold but does not last very long' (trigeminal neuralgia)
- 'Jaw pain, really tight and aching when I wake up in the morning and when I get stressed at work' (TMD)
- 'It feels like my mouth is burning and it's all the time' (burning mouth syndrome)
- 'A constant throbbing and aching pain where my tooth was extracted months ago but my dentist said everything looks OK' (atypical odontalgia).

2.5.2 **When did you first notice the pain? What do you believe caused it?**

A known trigger or event at the time of pain onset can be helpful in the diagnosis. Obtain details on any trauma, illness or infection, dental or surgical treatment, stressful life event, or did it 'just happen'. For example:

- 'Pain started after my jaw was kept wide open for a long time when the impacted wisdom teeth were removed' (possible temporomandibular joint damage)
- 'Occurred after an attack of shingles' (postherpetic neuralgia, neuropathic pain).

2.5.3 **Temporal quality and pain duration**

For example:

- Brief sharp episodes of pain lasting seconds to a few minutes in trigeminal neuralgia
- Pain episodes lasting for several hours on awakening from nocturnal bruxism in TMD
- Constant pain, i.e. never free from pain but does vary in intensity in neuropathic pain.

2.5.4 **Pain intensity**

Pain intensity does not provide any information on the diagnosis but allows for a rapid measurement of the progress of treatment by compiling a daily or weekly 'usual' pain intensity score. In addition, having the patient complete 'minimum' and 'maximum' intensity scores over the last week or month in conjunction with relieving and aggravating modalities is helpful in constructing the pain management plan. More detail on how this can be measured can be

Figure 2.2 Taking a pain history

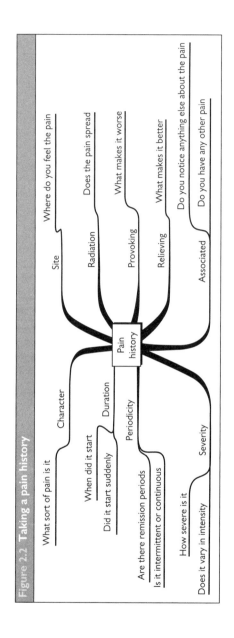

Pain history

Site
Where do you feel the pain
Radiation
Does the pain spread

Provoking
What makes it worse

Relieving
What makes it better

Associated
Do you notice anything else about the pain
Do you have any other pain

Character
What sort of pain is it

Duration
When did it start
Did it start suddenly

Periodicity
Are there remission periods
Is it intermittent or continuous

Severity
How severe is it
Does it vary in intensity

found in Chapter 3. Modalities to be assessed include pain better or worse from rest, weather changes, heat, cold, pressure, touch, stress, being occupied, or medication. For example: 'My pain has varied between 2 and 7 over the month. It is 2 when I am busy and see my friends, but it is 7 when I get stressed' suggesting the pain management focus should be with psychological strategies such as cognitive behavioural therapy.

2.5.5 **Pain word descriptors**

Words and questionnaires describing the quality of pain such as the McGill Pain Questionnaire (see Chapter 3) are valuable and provide a global insight into the 'pain problem'. Sensory words give information on likely pathophysiology (e.g. 'shooting' neuralgic pain, 'cramping' myofascial pain, 'burning' neuropathic pain) while affective words illustrate the psychological aspect (e.g. 'sickening and fearful'). The intensity of the descriptor (mild, moderate or severe) is helpful in determining clinical treatment priorities, e.g. severe stabbing and shooting pain suggests an antineuralgic drug trial. However, a patient with mild cramping pain but severe fearful and punishing pain warrants a psychological priority.

2.5.6 **Location of pain**

Obtain information on both the original site of pain and to where it is spreading. Diagrams such as in Figure 2.3 can be completed by patients.

The anatomical areas to be considered: intraoral, extraoral, head and neck, and body pain sites (including abdominal and pelvic pain). Other questions to be asked include:

- Is the pain site discrete and unchanged? (e.g. unilateral condylar osteoarthritis)
- Is the pain spreading? suggesting peripheral/CNS neuronal plasticity or secondary myofascial pain
- Are there concurrent overlapping pain entities that require separate diagnostic terms and treatments? (e.g. migraine and TMD)
- Are there other symptoms associated in the pain area such as numbness, tingling, swelling, altered sensation? (suggestive of neuropathic trigeminal pain)
- Are there new pains requiring a diagnosis? For example, the recent onset of an acute pulpitis pain within an existing neuropathic pain area, i.e. the need to maintain routine dental examinations during chronic pain management in order to avoid masking a genuine positive response in treating chronic pain.
- Is there widespread body pain influencing orofacial pain, e.g. fibromyalgia and TMD?
- Is there a correlation in a change in pain intensity between orofacial and pelvic pain in the female cycle suggesting oestrogen-modulated pain? Conditions that vary with the menstrual cycle include memory, mood disorders, epilepsy, migraine and TMD.

Figure 2.3 Pain diagrams

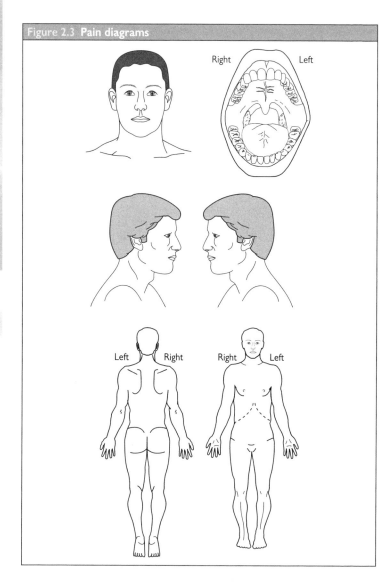

2.6 **Medical history**

2.6.1 **General history**

A detailed medical history should included heart/vasculature, respiratory, immune and endocrine systems, kidney and liver, skin and oral mucosa, infectious diseases/cancer, peripheral/CNS disorders, and with a particular emphasis on psychiatric and gastrointestinal problems.

2.6.2 **Specific questions**

- Is there comorbid anxiety/depression? These prolong and increase pain. If severe depression and anxiety is identified these factors are often a higher priority for treatment ahead of pain management.
- Are gastrointestinal problems likely to interfere or result with planned medication? Certain first-line antineuropathic drugs such as amitriptyline may increase the severity of pre-existing gastrointestinal disorders.
- Has the patient lost weight due to depression or increased weight from physical deconditioning or as a result of an amitriptyline side effect?
- How many other doctors, dentists and specialists have been consulted? Is the patient complaining of 'pain illiterate' doctors and dentists unable to formulate a correct diagnosis? Or is it due to a patient with unrealistic expectations: 'I have had the pain for 20 years but want a 100% pain reduction to move ahead with my life'. Is the patient a doctor 'shopper' and abuser of the health system?

2.6.3 **Medical, dental and allied health treatments**

Before prescribing any drugs it is essential to find out more about the past treatment history and these are summarized in Figure 2.4.

Treatments will include:

- Medical: medication, surgery
- Dental: root canal therapy, oral surgery, occlusal splint, adjusting occlusion
- Allied health: acupuncture, chiropractic, herbs, hypnosis, biofeedback, yoga and meditation, osteopathy, physiotherapy, psychological counselling, spiritual healing and prayer.

2.7 **Psychological assessment**

This is essential and further details are provided in Chapter 3.

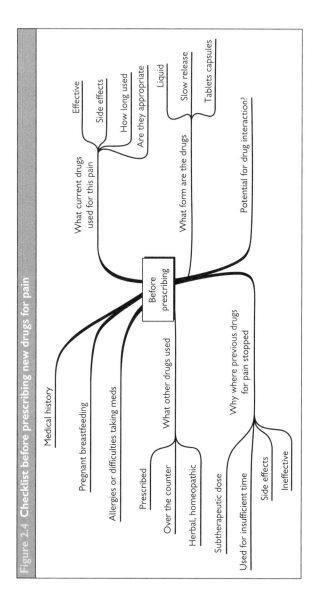

Figure 2.4 Checklist before prescribing new drugs for pain

2.8 **Social/environmental assessment**

The main features are summarized in Table 2.2

2.8.1 **Effect of pain on employment, social activities and sleep**

Distress associated with intense pain is likely to be amplified where pain 'interferes' with the satisfactory performance of everyday roles and activities. A major mediating variable is a cognitive appraisal on the part of the patient that many important aspects of their daily life are no longer under their control.

2.8.2 **Frequency and nature of contact with health professionals regarding pain**

Some people with chronic facial pain consult a remarkable number of health professionals over a long period of time. When a course of treatment fails to satisfy their expectations, which may be quite unrealistic, the patient suffers frustration and perhaps anger, increasing autonomic activity and dysphoria, and reducing compliance with disability-reduction regimes. A process of demoralization occurs over time.

2.8.3 **Patient's beliefs of the cause of his or her pain**

It is essential to determine these as these will influence response to treatment. The most common one is that the pain is a sign of something more sinister. Many also think that the pain will get worse especially if they overuse the area.

2.8.4 **Patient's and family's expectations from treatment**

Patient expectations are cognitive variables that need to be identified early in the pain assessment interview so information can be provided. Based on a long frustrating history of incorrect diagnoses and failed treatments, patients attending a pain clinic initially admit that they expect the treatment from the clinic will have no effect on their pain problem. Thus, low or negative expectations of help can be frequently associated with an ongoing search for help.

Table 2.2 Social history
• School & childhood: overall assessment, lonely, history of bullying, truant, illness, relationships
• Education: level of education, satisfaction
• Work including housework and satisfaction: previous posts, present, stress factors
• Leisure activity: how relax physical, cognitive, alone, team activities
• Marital status: past and present, stress factors
• Children: number, ages, problems, worries
• Finance: worries
• Housing: type, quality, satisfaction.

2.9 **Examination**

Pain is an invisible symptom and cannot be observed by a clinical examination. A standardized approach to the physical examination process is conducted to identify pathology as a possible (co-)causal factor of pain. The regional examination should be performed with visual inspection, palpation, percussion and auscultation.

- Facial expression and pain behaviour
- Examination of face including vascular changes, tumours, signs of trauma, oedema, eyes, sinuses, neck and salivary glands
- Neurological examination and in particular cranial nerve examination – see Table 2.3
- Mental state – may be necessary with some patients
- Hard tissues and teeth – for obvious dental pathology including excessive wear facets indicating bruxism, inadequate occlusion, fixed and removal appliances.
- Oral mucosa – for soft tissue lesions
- Musculature – muscles of mastication, head and neck muscles for tenderness and trigger points, muscle hypertrophy, limitation and restriction.
- TMJ – for crepitus, limited or excessive jaw movements, capsular and meniscal pathology or discrepancy, condylar hyper-/hypoplasia.
- Spinal pathologies affecting dorsal roots of C2-4 innervating the angle of the mandible.
- Exclusion of headache syndromes and CNS/brain pathology.

Table 2.3 Cranial nerve examination

Nerve	Number	Function and testing
Olfactory	I	Smell using several different smells
Optic	II	Visual acuity, papillary light responses, visual fields, fundoscopy
Oculomotor	III	Ocular movements, diplopia
Trochlear	IV	Light reaction, ocular movement
Trigeminal	V	Sensation of the face, muscles of mastication: corneal reflex, light touch, pin prick , strength of muscles of mastication, jaw jerk
Abducens	VI	Ocular movements, diplopia
Facial	VII	Muscles of facial expression: frown, eye closure, smile, pouting
Acoustic	VIII	Hearing whisper, watch, Rinne's and Weber test, Nystagmus
Glossophayngeal	IX	Gag reflex applied to tonsillar fossa
Vagal	X	Palatal elevation during phonation, vocal cord function
Accessory	XI	Elevation of shoulder, neck rotation with/without resistance
Hypoglossal	XII	Deviation of tongue, fasciculation, wasting

2.10 **Conclusion**

Anyone with an abnormal history and examination will need either further investigation or referral to other specialists. In the books listed below you will find examples of how this data could be recorded on semi-structured forms.

2.11 **References**

Bird, J., Cohen-Cole, S.A. (1990). The three-function model of the medical interview. An educational device. *Advances in Psychosomatic Medicine*, **20**: 65–88.

Drangsholt, M., Truelove, E. (2001). Trigeminal neuralgia mistaken as temporomandibular disorder. *Journal Evidence Based Dental Practise*, **1**: 41–50.

Rudy, T.E. and Turk, D.C. (1991). Psychological aspects of pain. *International Anesthesiology Clinics*, **29**: 9–21.

Turk, D.C. (1990). Customizing treatment for chronic pain patients: who, what, and why. *Clinical Journal of Pain*, **6**: 255–70.

Vickers, E.R. and Boocock, H. (2005). Chronic orofacial pain is associated with psychological morbidity and negative personality changes: a comparison to the general population. *Australian Dental Journal*, **50**: 21–30.

Vickers, E.R. (2005). *Orofacial pain: problem based learning*. Sydney University Press.

Zakrzewska, J.M. (2002). Chapter 4, History taking, and Chapter 5, Examination, in Zakrzewska, J.M., Harrison, S.D., ed *Assessment and management of orofacial pain*. pp 51–85. Elsevier, Amsterdam.

24

Chapter 3

Investigations

Peter Svensson, Lene Baad-Hansen, Toby Newton-John,
Suk Ng, and Joanna M. Zakrzewska

> **Key points**
>
> - Investigations need to be ordered in the light of the clinical findings and then interpreted again using the clinical findings
> - Blood tests may be required in order to exclude certain diagnoses or for monitoring purposes
> - A variety of neurophysiological tests can be performed but many are not in routine clinical use
> - Imaging should be done after careful consideration
> - There are a variety of dental images that can be used to rule out dental causes for pain
> - CT and MRI have a role to play in facial pain diagnostics but mainly rule out carcinoma
> - The assessment of relevant psychological areas can be done quickly and without the need for specialized psychological knowledge. This assessment can improve treatment planning and therefore patient care significantly.

3.1 Chapter plan

Figure 3.1 is an outline of the main contents of this chapter.

3.2 Importance of investigations

Investigations are done to:
- Confirm or exclude a diagnosis
- Aid treatment planning
- Monitor treatment or outcome measures
- Monitor side effects or adverse reactions.

Figure 3.1 Chapter plan

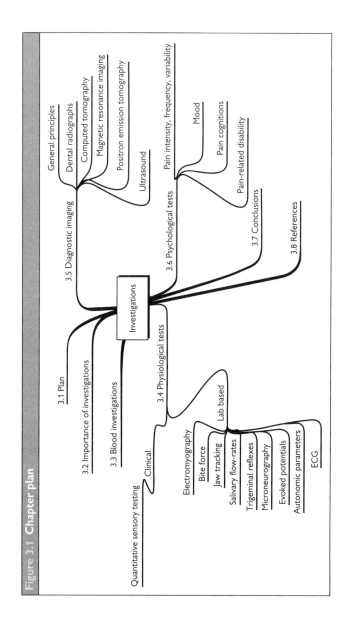

Many patients are often over-investigated because a careful history and examination have not been done and it is thought erroneously that the investigations will pick up everything. Sometimes unexpected results are obtained which then need to be interpreted not only in the light of the presenting complaint but also as possible unrelated factors. It has been shown that the highest number of abnormal results is found when the tests are deemed essential. Investigations need to be requested in the light of the clinical findings and then interpreted again using the clinical findings. There are relatively few investigations needed for facial pain patients and those which may be of relevance to facial pain are now going to be discussed.

3.3 **Blood investigations**

A variety of these may be done and some are important in order to rule out other diagnosis. These are shown in Figure 3.2.

Investigations of patients with burning mouths are important in order to rule out treatable causes and these are discussed further in Chapter 7 on burning mouth syndrome. It is important to rule out haematological abnormalities including malignant ones and so it is good practise to do a basic full blood count and differential count on all patients with facial pain. Patients with paroxysmal hemicrania may have a haemoglobinopathy and it is important to rule these out in patients who are to have surgery. In first division trigeminal pain vasculitis, for example, cranial arteritis remains an important differential and so an ESR is important. A C reactive protein test may also be helpful.

Disorders that may co-exist and may need to be investigated include:

• Trigeminal neuropathies and connective tissue disorders

• Depression and thyroid disease

• Multiple sclerosis and trigeminal neuralgia.

Some baseline and then monitoring tests are important when using certain drugs, e.g. white cell count, urea and electrolytes, liver function and folate with anticonvulsants. Patients on warfarin need to be monitored carefully especially if they are given carbamazepine.

Renal and liver functions may need to be tested if prescribed drugs are excreted through the kidneys or liver, both at baseline and at subsequent visits. Abnormal liver function tests due to drugs normally resolve within 3–4 weeks after withdrawal and if they do not then some form of liver disease or alcohol overuse may be accounting for them.

Drug levels are used for assessing compliance and in order to forecast toxicity. Drug levels are not used frequently with chronic facial pain, as there is often little need to check on adherence to therapy.

Table 3.1 presents some abnormal results and how they may be interpreted in the light of the diagnosis of facial pain.

Figure 3.2 Blood investigations done in facial pain patients

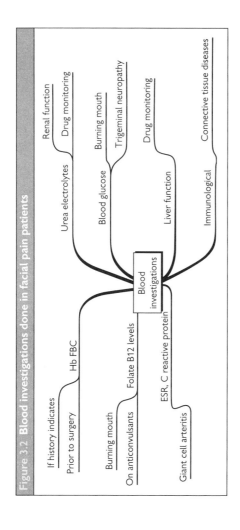

Table 3.1 Interpretation of results			
Test	**Abnormality**	**Possible diagnosis**	**Further evaluation**
Haemoglobin	Lowered	Anaemia, may be related to temporal arteritis, immunological disorders	Depends on other parameters
MCV and MCH	Raised	Vitamin B_{12}, folate deficiency potentially related to drug therapy Alcohol/liver disease	Serum vitamin B_{12}, red cell folate Liver function tests, thyroid function
MCV	Lowered	Chronic blood loss Iron deficiency aneamia Thalasseamia Drug induced	Blood film, serum ferritin, reticulocyte count, electrophoresis, faecal occult bloods
ESR	Raised	Elevated among others in patients with temporal artertis	Temporal artery biopsy
	Lowered	Iron deficiency aneamia, megaloblastic anaemia, thalassemia	
Gamma glutamyl transferase GGT	High	Liver disease, alcohol use, drug induced	
Alkaline phosphatase	High	Liver disease, gallstones, drug induced bone disease	GGT, isoenzymes to determine whether due to bony causes
Liver transaminases	High	Liver disease, thyroid disease, heart failure, drugs	
Autoanitobody screen – Anti-Ro and Anti-La, thyroid		Painful trigeminal neuropathies – Sjogren's syndrome, scleroderma Thyroid disease	Labial gland biopsy for Sjogrens Thyroid hormone levels

29

3.4 Physiological investigations

A comprehensive pain assessment should include measurements of spontaneous pain and stimulus-evoked pain. The assessment of spontaneous pain is discussed in section 3.6.

3.4.1 Clinical assessment of stimulus-evoked pain

This can be done with quantitative sensory testing (QST) and simple chair-side tests. In some orofacial pain conditions (e.g. neuropathic pain), there may be sensory deficits (hypoesthesia/hypoalgesia) or hyperphenomena (hyperalgesia/

allodynia). In the clinic, these phenomena can be tested by the use of standard dental or medical office equipment (see Table 3.2) Clinical assessment will normally use the patient's contralateral (non-painful) side as a control in the determination of whether there is a change in mechanical or thermal sensitivity (increased, decreased, normal). If changes in sensitivity are present, it is useful to map the affected areas of skin or mucosa, for example for follow-up purposes for patients with nerve damage.

Pressure algometers can quantify the degree of mechanical sensitization and can serve as an additional measurement to palpation.

3.4.2 **Laboratory tests**

3.4.2.1 *Electromyography (EMG)*

EMG is used for the measurement of muscle activity by recording action potentials (electrical signals) from muscle fibres when they contract. Electromyographic recordings of jaw muscle activity can be useful in orofacial pain cases where abnormalities in muscle activity are suspected, for example in cases with facial asymmetry with a possibility of muscular hypertrophy or atrophy and in patients with involuntary muscle contractions (dystonia).

3.4.2.2 *Bite force*

Maximum bite force evaluation is a fairly simple procedure which is mostly used for research purposes, however, it can useful for assessment of degenerative muscle disorders, e.g. myasthenia gravis or bulbar myasthenia gravis.

3.4.2.3 *Jaw tracking*

The diagnostic value of jaw tracking for measurement of the mandibular range of motion in patients with orofacial pain has been under debate. It is a technique by which the movements of the lower jaw can be measured in three dimensions. It requires a jaw tracking device and is mostly used for research purposes. No immediate diagnostic benefit is obtained which cannot be achieved with a simple metal ruler.

3.4.2.4 *Salivary flow-rates*

Stimulated and unstimulated salivary flow-rates can be evaluated for whole saliva or individually for the parotid or sublingual/submandibular glands by sialometry. The simplest technique is measurement of unstimulated whole saliva.

Table 3.2 Clinical physiological tests		
Test	**Fibres**	**Method**
touch	Aβ-fibres	cotton swab lightly stroking across the skin or mucosa
punctuate stimuli	mainly Aδ-fibres	pricking with a blunt needle or a toothpick
cold	mainly Aδ-fibres	cool metal object
heat	C-fibres	warm metal object

The unstimulated salivary flow rate test 'draining method' consists of:

- No eating or drinking for at least 90 minutes prior to collection
- Patient told not to move tongue, lips, cheeks, etc.
- Patient to sit in a relaxed position and saliva allowed to run into a plastic cup for 10–15 minutes
- Salivary flow rate is calculated as ml/min.

Stimulation of salivary flow can be obtained by letting the patient chew 1 g of paraffin during collection. These tests are useful in cases where hyposalivation is suspected if patients complain of xerostomia or Sjögren's Syndrome is suspected.

3.4.2.5 *Trigeminal reflexes*

Trigeminal reflexes, like the blink reflex, have been suggested to serve as an objective measure of orofacial pain. These reflexes are modulated by experimental pain and can be altered in some orofacial pain conditions, indicating a connection between trigeminal reflex circuits and nociceptive pathways. Furthermore, EMG recordings of reflex responses involving the trigeminal nerve among others can be useful when neural damage or disease is suspected. For the evaluation of orofacial pain, however, these techniques show low sensitivity, specificity, and prognostic values, however, they can be helpful in the differential diagnosis of structural lesions in the brainstem, e.g. due to stroke.

3.4.2.6 *Microneurography*

This is a technically demanding method, which allows for single-fibre recording from nerve fibres in awake subjects. It can be used for the determination of physiological characteristics of different classes of nerve fibres but the technique cannot be used in a standard clinical setting. Compound action potentials can be recorded from both the mandibular and maxillary nerve and will indicate the functional integrity of the peripheral nerve segment.

3.4.2.7 *Evoked potentials*

The functional integrity of the trigemino-cortical pathways can be assessed with somatosensory-evoked cortical potentials. They are relevant if structural lesions are suspected in the central nociceptive pathways (stroke, disseminated sclerosis, etc) but will not be relevant for most orofacial pain conditions.

3.4.2.8 *Autonomic parameters*

Autonomic parameters such as heart rate, blood pressure, sweat secretion, and temperature are coupled to pain but are too multifactorial so are not used in a standard clinical evaluation of orofacial pain.

3.4.2.9 *ECG*

Electrocardiographic monitoring may be useful for facial pain associated with autonomic features and glossopharyngeal neuralgia in order to detect cardiac arrythmias. These may occur during attacks of pain.

3.5 **Diagnostic Imaging**

3.5.1 **General principles**

Diagnostic imaging is integral to the clinical management of many types of disease. However, techniques which use X-rays pose potential cancer risks for patients and staff. The International Commission on Radiological Protection (ICRP) recommends that imaging should only be done if there is a net positive benefit for the patient, and all exposures should be kept as low as reasonably practicable.

Pain in the orofacial region does not automatically require X-ray imaging. However, when a clinical history and examination has revealed some possible differential diagnoses, then imaging may be of value either to confirm or exclude a diagnosis. Each imaging modality has certain clinical indications and all imaging have some drawbacks.

The circumstances where radiological investigations may not be required are:

- Most TMJ problems are due to soft tissue dysfunction rather than bony changes, and soft tissues do not show up on X-ray imaging. In the UK, national guidelines discourage X-rays for TMJ problems. However, in some countries there seems to be a prerequisite, perhaps for insurance purposes, to exclude bony pathology in the condyles and panoramic radiographs almost become the norm. Any bony changes which do take place tend to appear late and are often absent in the acute phase, hence X-ray imaging does not add any useful information which might influence the diagnosis or patient management

- In patients with chronic idiopathic facial pain it is important before taking new radiographs to collect and examine carefully all existing radiographs, especially if the patient has already had common dental diseases such as pulpitis investigated and ruled out. Rarely are more investigations required

- Radiography for sinus disease is not indicated as acute sinusitis can be diagnosed and treated clinically. Signs on X-ray sinus are often non-specific and are encountered in asymptomatic people.

3.5.1.1 *Digital radiography*

Digital radiographs, being electronically stored rather than directly exposed on film, can be e-mailed or otherwise duplicated electronically. They are easily passed on to other clinicians thus precluding unnecessary repeat radiation dosage to the patient.

A variety of images are used in investigation of orofacial pain. Table 3.3 lists the main images that are used for investigation of orofacial pain and provides some indications for their use.

3.5.2 **Dental radiographs**

Radiography is a standard technique for assessing dental health and disease. Research has shown that intraoral (bitewing and periapical) radiography is

Type of Imaging	Indications	Interpretation/what would be seen
Table 3.3 Indications for diagnostic imaging in orofacial pain		
Intra-oral radiographs		
Periapical	Chronic periapical abscess	Radiolucency in bone surrounding root apex
Periapical	Periodontal abscess	Increased size of periodontal ligament space
Bitewing	Caries	Radiolucency in enamel and/or dentine
Occlusal	Alternative to periapical if latter not possible, submandibular salivary stone	Radio opacity in area of duct
Extraoral radiographs		
Dental panoramic tomography	Chronic periapical abscesses in more than one quadrant	Radiolucency in bone surrounding root apices of several teeth
Dental panoramic tomography	TMJ ankylosis	Bony union between condyle and glenoid fossa; no radiolucent joint space
Oblique lateral	Alternative to DPT if latter not possible	
Contrast studies		
Sialography	Salivary stone (meal time syndrome)	Stone may be radiopaque if calcified, salivary ducts proximal to stone are dilated and may have sausage-linking appearance
Arthrography	TMJ internal derangement of disc	Contrast medium filling lower ± upper joint space, indirectly showing outline of disc
Specialised imaging		
Computed tomography (CT)	Chronic sinusitis requiring surgery	Thickened mucosal lining, obstruction of ostium
CT	TMJ ankylosis	Malformation of condyle and glenoid fossae. Loss of joint space.
Magnetic resonance imaging (MRI)	TMJ internal derangement of disc, especially where surgery is being planned	Disc differentiated from surrounding tissues, in pseudo-dynamic function
MRI	Suspected cancer	Space occupying lesion ± invasion of adjacent tissues
MRI	Trigeminal neuralgia	Plaques of multiple sclerosis, neoplasia, AV malformations, compressions of nerve
Bone Scintigraphy	Suspected cancer affecting bone	Hot spots in affected bone and maybe metastases elsewhere in skeleton
Ultrasound	Salivary stone (meal time syndrome)	Stone appears as bright white line with distal acoustic shadow, gland may show abnormal echotexture
	Swelling in soft tissue e.g. infected sebaceous cyst; tumour	Space occupying lesion with different echogenicity to surrounding tissues

superior to panoramic radiography for the diagnosis of common dental pathology (caries, periodontal and periapical pathology). Figure 3.3 shows a bitewing with caries and Figure 3.4 shows a periapical with a lesion at the apex.

Figure 3.3 Bitewing with caries

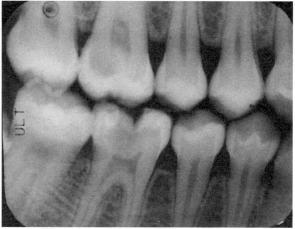

Bitewing radiograph showing occlusal caries in upper and lower right first molars. The occlusal enamel is clearly perforated in the lower tooth but still intact in the upper (occult caries). The former is easy to diagnose clinically but the latter is more challenging. Both teeth would give chronic dental pain.

Figure 3.4 Periapical with a lesion at the apex

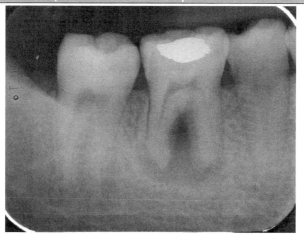

Periapical radiograph showing radiolucent area at apices and inter-radicular region of lower right first molar. Apices are resorbed. This is a large chronic periapical abscess.

In cases of irreversible pulpitis the corresponding changes in bone architecture may not be radiographically detectable for 2 weeks, thus a repeat radiograph may be necessary. A panoramic radiograph covers a much larger area for both jaws than an intraoral radiograph and is useful where a bony lesion is not fully shown on the latter. This is seen in Figure 3.5.

If bone disease such as ankylosis or arthritis is suspected, then a panoramic radiograph would be able to provide a gross assessment of the condyles and glenoid fossae. Radiographic examination is also indicated where there is recent evidence of progressive pathology such as change in occlusion, sensory or motor alterations, change in range of movement. Some panoramic machines have a special TMJ programme which allow views of left and right TMJ in mouth open and closed positions ('4-in-1' view).

3.5.3 Computed tomography CT

This is used in a variety of situations and can be used with a contrast medium in order to increase their potential including:

- Sinus disease – can be used in sinus disease which has failed to resolve after 10 days and also when it is necessary to show the presence and distribution of disease and sinonasal anatomy before functional endoscopic sinus surgery. A low-dose radiation technique should be used. CT is indicated when maximum medical treatment is ineffective. Contrast-enhanced CT (with coronal and axial images) are specialized investigations indicated when there is development of complications such as orbital cellulitis, or if malignancy is suspected

- TMJ – may be useful in special circumstances such as post-surgical repair, implants or bony ankylosis. Figure 3.6 shows the coronal and axial views of the TMJ with ankylosis

- Recent onset and rapidly increasing frequency and severity of headache, headache causing patient to wake from sleep; associated dizziness, lack of coordination, tingling or numbness; headache made worse by coughing, sneezing or straining are some of the indications

35

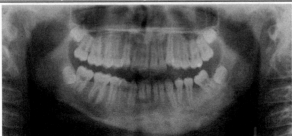

Figure 3.5 Dental panoramic tomograph

Dental panoramic tomograph (DPT) showing chronic diffuse sclerosing osteomyelitis in left mandible, together with periosteal reaction ('onion skin' layering at inferior border).

- Suspected carcinomas especially if invading bone
- Can be used to guide biopsies.

3.5.4 **Magnetic resonance imaging MRI**

- Used to determine if there is a carcinoma
- TMJ, with its superior demonstration of various soft tissues, is the investigation of choice to identify internal disk derangement, especially if surgery is being planned
- Trigeminal neuralgia for determination of AV malformations, tumours, multiple sclerosis, compression of the nerve.

Figure 3.6 Coronal and axial views of TMJ with ankylosis

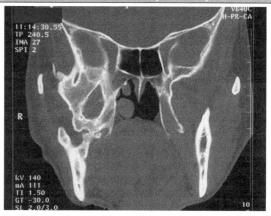

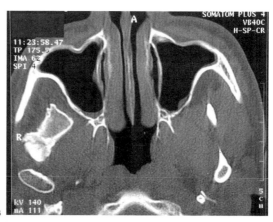

Coronal (A) and axial (B) CT images of patient with ankylosis of right TMJ. Note enlarged and misshapen condyle and base of skull on affected side. Axial image (B) shows enlarged right coronoid process, compared to normal left coronoid.

Figure 3.7 shows a tumour on the trigeminal nerve.

Table 3.4 shows the advantages and disadvantages of MRI and CT.

3.5.5 Positron emission tomography (PET)

Using nuclear medicine techniques a three-dimensional image or map of functional processes in the body can be produced. It can be used alongside CT and MRI but is expensive and not in wide clinical use at present. Its primary role is to demonstrate carcinoma and any recurrences. It is increasingly being used for imaging brain function.

3.5.6 Ultrasound

Ultrasound imaging is considered to be first line investigation of swellings in soft tissue. It will identify the organ or tissue of origin and differentiate cystic from solid lesions. It is invaluable in imaging the salivary glands and problems such as salivary stones. Ultrasound imaging may help show an effusion in TMJ but has not been fully evaluated.

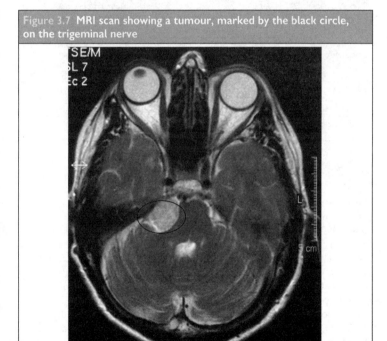

Figure 3.7 **MRI scan showing a tumour, marked by the black circle, on the trigeminal nerve**

Table 3.4 Use of computed tomography (CT) magnetic resonance imaging (MRI) in facial pain

Characteristic	CT	MRI
Radiation dose	High	None
Organs and tissues shown	Excellent bone detail. Poor to moderate soft tissue detail. Blood vessels shown if inject contrast medium	Excellent soft tissue detail, especially brain. Poor detail of bone, teeth and air. Blood vessels shown if use special echo sequence – magnetic resonance angiography (MRA)
Availability	Widely available in many hospitals in many countries	Expensive. Available but not as widely as CT
Presence of metal fixtures, e.g. dental amalgams	Produces artefacts (less on modern machines)	May produce some artifact
Presence of loose metal fragments and certain types of surgical clips inside the patient	Produces artefacts but still can have CT done	May move when in magnetic field and cause internal injury or haemorrhage – may contraindicate MRI
Cardiac pacemaker	Not affected by CT	Contraindicate MRI
Effect of patient movement	May not affect image if only minor movements	Will cause severe movement artefacts – patient must be able to keep still for many minutes
Scan time	Several to tens of minutes depending on site and detail required	Up to an hour or more depending on complexity
Patient experience	Relatively easily accepted, quiet, spacious	Can be claustrophobic and very noisy

3.6 **Psychological investigations**

The experience of unremitting pain is distressing in and of itself. We never expect to experience pain long term, and more severe pain is usually considered to represent a more sinister underlying pathology, creating additional anxiety and fear. When the body fails to heal itself, or the medical system fails to rid us of what hurts us, the psychological sequelae can be significant. Clearly the experience of persistent pain does not occur in a vacuum, and the individual's pre-existing psychological 'make up' will impact on how he or she responds to the stressor that is chronic pain.

Psychological disturbance in patients with chronic pain is high with depression running as high as 50% and anxiety disorders such as Post Traumatic Stress Disorder estimated as high as 15% in chronic orofacial pain. Less formal assessment of chronic orofacial pain group show high levels of anger, fear, distress and frustration when compared to a non-pain control group.

Carrying out some form of psychological assessment or screening of patients presenting with persistent orofacial pain should be a mandatory element of the treatment work up. A large number of rapidly administered, easily comprehensible self-report inventories exist which provide information about many important aspects of the chronic pain experience. Most questionnaires do not require any specialized psychological training to interpret. Items are usually summed, and the total score is compared to normative data to determine to what extent a given patient is 'deviating' from the average in his or her responding.

Patients can be given a questionnaire booklet to complete prior to their initial evaluation which contains:

• Demographic information

• Current medications and treatments

• Self-report questionnaires.

Although this may run to several pages and take some time to complete, clinicians should not be dissuaded by this. Patients who are not prepared to make this effort as part of their evaluation process are not likely to be motivated when it comes to their treatment.

Many hundreds of different self-report questionnaires have been developed in order to assess all aspects of the pain experience, and often there is little to recommend one questionnaire over another, other than personal preference. However, there are a number of assessment domains that should be given consideration when compiling a psychological investigation battery, as shown in Table 3.5.

Table 3.5 A selection of psychological tests to use in orofacial pain

Domain	Test	Scoring	Significant result
Pain intensity	Verbal rating scale Visual analogue scale	Score 0–10 Score 0–10	>4 mm >4 mm
Pain character	McGill pain Questionnaire long and/or short	Pain rating index Number of words chosen	>19 on total score short form McGill
Mood	Beck depression inventory Depression anxiety stress scale Hospital anxiety and depression scale	21 items scoring 0–3 42 items in total; 14 in each subscale 14 items, 7 in each subscale	>2–3 on suicide item, >20 on total score >14 on depression subscale >10 on either anxiety depression
Cognitions	Pain Catastrophizing Scale Pain Self Efficacy Questionnaire	13 items 10 items in total, scored 0–60	>30 tendency to catastrophise <12 low confidence >40 high confidence
Pain related disability	Multidimensional Pain Inventory Brief Pain Inventory Oral health impact	Each subscale is scored on a 0–6 scale Scale of 0–10 on a variety of parameters 14 items in total	Depends on subscale used >4 mm >25

3.6.1 **Pain intensity, frequency, variability**

Having a pre-treatment evaluation of pain intensity is obviously important for treatment monitoring, and a simple 0 to 10 numerical rating scale, anchored by 'no pain' at one end and 'pain as bad as it can be' at the other, is a valid and reliable measure. It should be clear that the evaluation is of averaged pain levels (perhaps over the last week is a realistic time frame) rather than current pain levels. Visual analogue scales can also be used, whereas more sophisticated pain intensity measures such as the widely used McGill Pain Questionnaire require more time for completion and scoring but providing additional qualitative information which may be particularly relevant for a chronic orofacial pain population (i.e. descriptor endorsement of pain as 'shooting', 'burning', 'stabbing', or 'aching' may have diagnostic value).

3.6.2 **Mood**

Patients presenting with marked elevations in depression, anxiety, or general distress are not likely to respond to their pain treatment; and failure to improve the pain symptoms will only contribute further to their psychological distress. An evidence based approach to questionnaires used to detect depression has suggested that the specificity and sensitivity of two questions as shown in Table 3.6 may be sufficient to alert the clinician that there is a mood disturbance.

Many self-report inventories have been developed in order to assess mood disorders:

- The Beck Depression Inventory has items on suicidal ideation and helplessness, and these should be inspected closely. Any patient scoring 2 or 3 on the suicidal thinking item, or more than 20 in total score, should be referred for clinical psychology or psychiatric evaluation
- The Depression Anxiety Stress Scale (DASS) is a newer measure with a number of advantages: three subscales are provided, there is a 21-item short form with excellent psychometrics, there are good normative data available using chronic pain samples, and it is freely available on the web (http://www2.psy.unsw.edu.au/groups/dass//)

The Hospital Anxiety and Depression scale was developed many years ago to assist non psychiatrists working in out-patient settings to determine whether their patients were at risk of anxiety or depression. There are 14 questions – seven on each topic and scores above 10 indicate that depression or anxiety may be present.

Table 3.6 Key questions to detect depression
• During the past month have you often been bothered by feeling down, depressed or hopeless?
• During the past month have you often be bothered by having little interest or pleasure in doing things?
• If patients answer yes to either question then the specificity of screening can be further increased by asking them whether they want help with their problems

3.6.3 **Pain cognitions**

Catastrophizing, or the tendency to interpret an event in the most negative or pessimistic way possible, has been documented in recent years as highly relevant to coping with persistent pain problems. Pain patients who catastrophize about their pain (e.g. 'this pain is overwhelming', 'there is nothing I can do about my pain', 'this pain will never get any better') do less well from any kind of treatment and it is strongly correlated with elevations in distress. The Pain Catastrophizing Scale assesses the frequency of such thoughts in relation to the pain problem.

At the other end of the cognitive spectrum, self-efficacy refers to the belief that one has the capability of undertaking a specific action successfully. The Pain Self Efficacy Questionnaire asks patients to rate how confident they are that they could carry out various day to day activities (paid employment, socialize, make plans, etc) despite pain. It is a very useful clinical tool, not only to determine patient confidence in their pain management, but also as an outcome measure following treatment. Patients scoring less than 12 are at risk of treatment drop out because their confidence is so low. Those scoring 40 or above are in the range associated with attending work reliably despite chronic pain, and this makes a useful benchmark.

3.6.4 **Pain-Related Disability/Pain Limitations**

While there are many such assessment instruments in the general chronic pain field, the sensitivity of these general measures to detect the physical limitations associated with orofacial pain is lacking. The Multidimensional Pain Inventory has been applied to temporomandibular joint disorders and has a wealth of normative data available. A much less onerous measure is the ten item Brief Pain Inventory where the patient rates the extent to which pain interferes with life areas such as sleep, work, relations with others and enjoyment of life. For facial pain in particular, the Oral Health Impact Profile was developed and contains items relating to social anxiety (eating, smiling, and talking in public) which are commonly affected in this patient group.

3.7 **Conclusions**

Investigations need to be used with care and some still remain research based and have not been evaluated for their sensitivity, specificity and predictive value. This is especially relevant to the physiological tests that are described.

The goal of including psychological factors as part of the investigation process is not to make a psychiatric diagnosis. It is:

• To introduce the patient to the biopsychosocial model of pain – education that thoughts, feelings and behaviours are just as important to the pain experience as the state of body tissues and their functions

- To identify whether there are potential psychosocial barriers to the effective treatment of the pain problem which require further investigation by a clinical psychologist or psychiatrist.

3.8 **References**

Anonymous (2007). *Making the best use of clinical radiology services. Referral Guidelines.* The Royal College of Radiologists, London. 6th edition.

Anonymous (2004). *Selection criteria for dental radiography. FGDP (UK) Good Practice Guidelines.* Faculty of General Dental Practitioners (UK), The Royal College of Surgeons of England. 2nd edition.

Beck, A.T., Ward, C.H., Mendelson, M., Mock, J. and Erbaugh, J. (1961). An inventory for measuring depression. *Archives of General Psychiatry,* **4**: 561–1.

Cleeland, C. (1994). Brief pain inventory, short form. Pain Research Group, University of Wisconsin at Madison, In McCaffery, M., Passer, O. *Pain, clinical manual* (p. 61). St. Louis: CV Mosby, Inc.

Kerns, R.D., Turk, D.C. and Rudy, T. (1985). The West Haven-Yale Multidimensional Pain Inventory. *Pain,* **23**: 45–6.

Miles, T.S., Nauntofte, B., Svensson, P (Eds.) (2004). *Clinical Oral Physiology.* Quintessence Publishing Co. Ltd. Copenhagen.

Nicholas, M.K.N. (2007). The pain self-efficacy questionnaire: Taking pain into account. *European Journal of Pain,* **11**: 153–163.

Rushton, V.E., Horner, K. (1996). The use of panoramic radiology in dental practice. *Journal of Dentistry,* **24**:185–201.

Slade, G.D. (1997). Derivation and validation of a short-form oral health impact profile. *Community Dental Oral Epidemiology,* **25**: 284–90.

Sullivan, M.J.L., Bishop, S.R. and Pivik, J. (1995). The Pain Catastrophizing Scale: development and validation. *Psychological Assessment,* **7**: 524–32.

Svensson, P., Baad-Hansen, L., Thygesen, T., Juhl, G.I., Jensen, T.S. (2004). Overview on tools and methods to assess neuropathic trigeminal pain. *Journal Orofacial Pain,* **18**: 332–8.

Chapter 4

Classification and diagnosis of orofacial pain

Joanna M. Zakrzewska and Jeffrey Okeson

Key points

- Correct diagnosis is the key to management of facial pain
- The diagnostic process involves several key steps: history, exam, analysis of findings, establishment of differential diagnosis, investigations, confirmation of diagnosis
- There are several classification systems for head and face pain
- Facial pain can be classified into three major groups which often dictate referral pathways
- Dental and oral mucosal pain disorders
- Musculoskeletal pain which mainly consist of temporomandibular pain (TMD)
- Neurovascular pain disorders which include neuropathic pain, neurovascular pain, other unclassifiable condition
- All patients with chronic facial pain will have psychological co-morbidity which in some cases will include depression and anxiety disorders.

43

4.1 Chapter plan

Figure 4.1 is an outline of the main contents of this chapter.

4.2 Introduction

The most critical task the clinician can provide for the patient is to establish the correct diagnosis. This is the foundation of successful treatment. Only after the correct diagnosis has been established can the proper treatment be selected. Establishing the correct diagnosis may also be the most difficult task for the clinician. Once a patient has acquired a diagnostic label it is difficult to change it so it is essential to take time over this aspect.

Figure 4.1 Plan for chapter

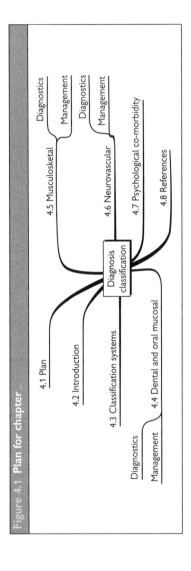

Figure 4.2 suggests the steps we need to go through in order to make the final diagnosis. In order to establish the proper diagnosis the clinician needs to acquire information from the following sources:

- Thorough history of the pain problem
- Thorough clinical examination of the patient
- Information from appropriate diagnostics test (i.e. images, blood studies)

Always be prepared to reconsider the diagnosis if:

- Patient fails to respond to the treatment that was suggested
- Condition worsens
- Clinical features no longer fit
- Oral cancer presents in a multitude of forms and always needs to be considered.

There are many different conditions that can produce orofacial pain. Some are simple and some are so complex they defy the experts.

4.3 **Classification systems**

The profession has developed several different classification schemes for these pain conditions, some based on the structures, some based on symptoms and others on treatments but all rely on expert opinion. The ones most relevant to head and neck pain patients are:

- International Association for the Study of Pain (IASP)
- International Headache Society (IHS)
- Research Diagnostic Criteria for Temporomandibular DIsorders (RDC/TMD).

However, the purpose of this chapter is not to elaborate in detail on each type of orofacial pain disorder. Instead it is to provide the general medical and dental practitioner with a basic guide to understanding, diagnosing, and managing orofacial pain disorders. Therefore, the classification used in this chapter will categorize orofacial pain disorders into three broad groups that will hopefully allow the practitioner to better direct the patient to the appropriate treatment options. Woda et al. have recently postulated that many of the orofacial diseases are in fact the same but because they arise from different tissues (bone, muscles, tooth, oral mucosa, joints) they are characterized differently. For more detailed descriptions of recent research in the area of classification of orofacial pain, the reader is referred to other sources. This is shown in Figure 4.3.

Figure 4.2 **Process for diagnosis**

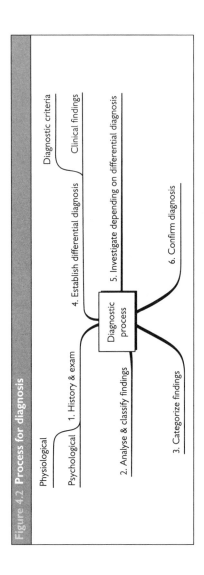

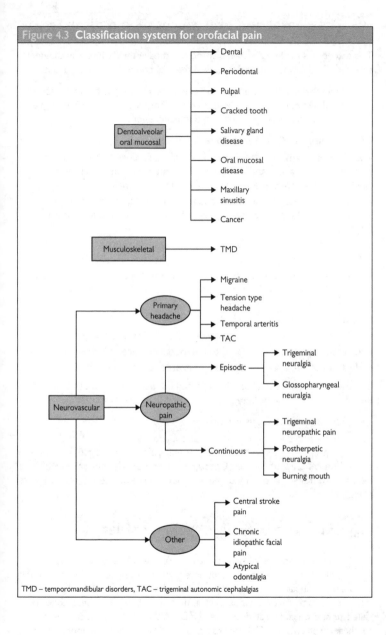

Figure 4.3 Classification system for orofacial pain

Dentoalveolar oral mucosal
→ Dental
→ Periodontal
→ Pulpal
→ Cracked tooth
→ Salivary gland disease
→ Oral mucosal disease
→ Maxillary sinusitis
→ Cancer

Musculoskeletal → TMD

Neurovascular
Primary headache
→ Migraine
→ Tension type headache
→ Temporal arteritis
→ TAC

Neuropathic pain
Episodic
→ Trigeminal neuralgia
→ Glossopharyngeal neuralgia

Continuous
→ Trigeminal neuropathic pain
→ Postherpetic neuralgia
→ Burning mouth

Other
→ Central stroke pain
→ Chronic idiopathic facial pain
→ Atypical odontalgia

TMD – temporomandibular disorders, TAC – trigeminal autonomic cephalalgias

4.4 **The dental and oral mucosal pain disorders**

This category is made up of pain disorders that have their sources in the dental structures and/or the mucosal tissues of the oral cavity. These will include:

(a) Dental: dental caries, pupal pain, dental abscesses, periodontal disease
(b) Oral mucosal lesions: lichen planus, aphthous stomatitis, herpes simplex, candidiasis, blistering conditions, traumatic lesions.

4.4.1 **Diagnostic Considerations**

The diagnostic key to identifying these pain disorders begins with listening carefully to the patient and an oral examination will often reveal the offending tooth or oral lesion. Some key features of dental pain include:

- The pain is located in the mouth and the pain is often increased by provocation of the structures, eating or biting down on the teeth increases the pain
- The particular tooth will often be identifying by the patient
- Temperature changes such as hot or cold liquids will greatly increase the pain
- If gingival and periodontal tissues are the source of pain these often appear inflamed and bleed easily to probing

Key features of oral mucosal lesions:

- Light touch to the lesion is painful
- Difficulty eating but not necessarily related to biting on a tooth
- Increase of pain is more related to the food substance contacting the lesion
- Heat or cold may also increase the pain, especially spicy foods.

In those cases when dental pain is suspected but not obvious upon examination, dental radiographs can be very helpful in establishing the diagnosis.

4.4.2 **Management Considerations**

This category of pain disorders is most appropriately managed in the dental office. Pupal pain disorders and periodontal pain are managed well by the general dental practitioner (see Chapter 6). When oral lesions are identified, a dentist with training in oral medicine is a good source of referral (see Chapters 6 and 7).

4.5 **The musculoskeletal pain disorders**

A very common source of orofacial pains are the musculoskeletal structures. The important structures to be considered are the muscles of mastication, the temporomandibular joints, and the associated structures such as ligament or tendons. Pains that have their sources in these structures have been collectively called temporomandibular disorders (TMD). Although many practitioners refer to these problems as 'TMJ' disorders, the joints are not the most common source of the pain. In fact, muscle pain is the most common type of TMD. Since the management of muscle pain is different than the management of joint pain, differentiating these conditions is an important task for the clinician.

4.5.1 Diagnostic Considerations

- TMD pain is often described as a dull, tight, achy pain
- Pain is most frequently felt in the preauricular areas over the temporomandibular joints
- It can be unilateral if one joint is involved or bilateral especially when muscle pain is the source
- Use of the masticatory system will increase the pain, thus pain is increased by eating, talking, yawning and singing
- Restricted mouth opening may be reported (normal mouth opening is consider to be 40 mm or greater between the anterior teeth)
- When an intracapsular condition is present there may be joint sounds noted during opening and closing
- Often the muscles of mastication, such as the masseter and temporal muscles, are tender or painful to palpation
- The TMJs may also be painful to palpate especially when the patient is asked to open and close
- Joint sounds can often be heard when the patient opens and closes the mouth and these may be associated with the pain complaint.

It should be noted that temporomandibular joint sounds are common in the general population and are not necessarily related to pain. Concern should arise when there is pain associated with the sounds or there are significant mechanical complaints present, such as, catching or locking of the joint.

4.5.2 Management Considerations

TMD pain disorders that are typically managed in the dental practice. Since there are a variety of etiologic factors associated with these conditions, their management is not always the same. In fact some of these conditions are simple to manage while others may take considerable effort. Patients who report a relatively mild, acute TMD may be referred to most general dental practitioners for management. In cases when the TMD symptoms are severe and chronic, more knowledgeable practitioners may need to be identified. Within the dental profession there are some practitioners who are selecting to specifically manage these conditions and a referral to one of these specially trained individuals is often a good choice (see Chapter 9).

4.6 Neurovascular orofacial pain disorders

Disorders in this category do not have their aetiologies in the dental or masticatory structures, even though the pain may be felt there. There are many of these pain disorders and grouping them into one category is not appropriate from a management stand point. However in this text this category is meant to help the practitioner separate the dental referrals from the medical referrals.

Within this category there are very common and well defined pain conditions felt in the orofacial structures. Such conditions are the primary headaches (i.e. migraine, tension-type), neuropathic pains (i.e. neuralgias, deafferentation) as well as pains originating from other structures of the head such as sinuses and ears. Many of these conditions will be elaborated upon in later chapters.

4.6.1 Diagnostic Considerations

It is important to remember that most of these conditions are not greatly influenced by provocation of the dental or masticatory structures. When jaw function does not greatly affect the pain, it is not likely dental, mucosal or musculoskeletal. Instead it is more likely a pain disorder that fits into this category.

Pain from these conditions may present in a variety of characteristics from constant to episodic, from mild to severe. Two of the most significant subcategories in this group are the neuropathic disorders and the neurovascular (migraine) disorders.

4.6.1.1 *Neuropathic pain disorders*

Neuropathic pain is characterized by pain felt in structures that have no clinical evidence of any pathology but follow a nerve distribution and can have the following features:

- The pain may be described as tingling, pins and needles like or have a burning quality
- Some of these pains will on occasion be sharp or electrical
- The pain is often increased disproportionally with mild stimulation
- The pain may be accompanied by other neurologic signs such as anaesthesia, paraesthesia, dysesthesia, hyperesthesia or hypoesthesia.
- Gross clinical examination is normal but sensory changes may be detected.

Episodic neuropathic pain disorders include trigeminal and glossopharyngeal neuralgia which are characterized by quick, intense, sharp, light touch provoked pains in the peripheral distribution of the affected nerve. It is usually momentary with complete remission of pain between episodes.

The trigeminal autonomic cephalgias which occur in the trigeminal region are often episodic but of longer duration than trigeminal neuralgia but most frequently in the first division. They are characterized by episodic pain with autonomic symptoms which can include tearing, eyelid oedema, nasal congestion, sweating and restlessness.

Continuous neuropathic pain which include post herpetic neuralgia, post traumatic neuralgias and burning mouth syndrome are characterized by fluctuations of pain intensity from high to low but they never completely resolve.

These are often characterized by tingling, burning pains in the distribution of a nerve branch/s. The patient may also describe numbness or sensations of crawling or itching (dysesthesia) in the painful area and sensory loss may be detected with careful testing.

4.6.1.2 *Neurovascular pain disorders*

Migraine is a neurovascular pain disorder which is characterized by severe yet benign pain typically presenting as a unilateral headache in the region of the eye and temple. A facial variant is also described in that the distribution is more in the second and third divisions. Migraines are episodic with typical durations of 4–8 hours. Between the episodes there is little to no headache. Patients will often report nausea and vomiting associated with the intense pain. Photophobia and phonophobia are common.

Temporal arteritis (giant cell arteritis) is a unilateral or bilateral headache of a continuous throbbing nature which is very intense. It often occurs in the elderly and is associated with tenderness and irregular shape of the temporal artery. Often associated with systemic symptoms and if not treated promptly can lead to blindness.

Tension headaches often become chronic and are described as continuous dull aching often symmetrical pain over the whole head extending down to the frontal area and they are not associated with any of the other features of migraine.

4.6.2 **Management Considerations**

Orofacial pain disorders in this category need to be managed medically. There may be a diagnostic problem since sometimes toothache is the patient's chief complaint (see Chapter 6) and patients do not realize that the pain originates from other structures. Neuropathic and neurovascular pain disorders are managed by directing therapies to the underlining pathophysiology and many respond dramatically to appropriate therapy (see Chapters 7, 10, 11 and 12).

Central causes such as post stroke pain and multiple sclerosis present rarely in the facial region. However pain will rarely be the primary symptom. Multiple sclerosis is closely linked with trigeminal neuralgia.

Patients who do not appear to fit into any category are often then labelled as atypical facial pain, now more frequently called chronic or persistent idiopathic facial pain or atypical odontalgia – if present in a very localized area. Some of these patients will probably be misdiagnosed as some form of neuropathic trigeminal pain (see Chapter 8).

4.7 **Psychological co-morbidity**

When a pain condition becomes more chronic, other influencing factors can further complicate and perpetuate the condition. Some of these factors may be psychological. These can include some of the following:

- Anxiety disorders, including posttraumatic stress
- Depression, a common mental disorder associated with chronic pain. Depression may be the result of the experience of chronic pain however on occasion depression may have resulted in the pain
- Personality traits, maladaptive health behaviours, hypochondrias and somatoform disorders may also be associated with chronic orofacial pain.

Each clinician should appreciate the influence of these factors and adequately assess them. Referral to the appropriate health care provider can be an essential part of management (see Chapter 5).

It has been proposed that a multiaxial approach should be taken to all pain patients whereby several parameters of illness are considered simultaneously and an appropriate scale for each parameter or axis is established. Thus patients have both a physiological diagnosis and a psychological one and it is the latter which may in some cases be more important for management than the physiological one. The psychological factors can change the whole approach to management and be the reason for non response to treatment.

4.8 **References**

Merskey, H., Bogduk, N. (1994). Classification of chronic pain. *Descriptors of Chronic Pain Syndromes and Definitions of Pain Terms.*, 2nd ed. Seattle: IASP Press.

Anonymous. (2004). Classification and diagnostic criteria for headache disorders, cranial neuralgias and facial pain. Headache Classification Committee of the International Headache Society. *Cephalalgia*, **24** (Suppl 1).

Okeson, J.P. (1996). *Orofacial pain guide: guidelines for assessment, diagnosis and management.* 1st ed. Chicago: Quintessence Publishing Company.

Dworkin, S.F., LeResche, L. (1992). Research diagnostic criteria for temporomandibular disorders: review, criteria, examinations and specifications, critique. *Journal Craniomandibular Disorders*, **6**: 301–55.

Turk, D.C., Rudy, T.E. (1992). Classification logic and strategies in chronic pain. In: Turk, D.C., Melzack, R., ed *Handbook of Pain Assessment*. New York: The Guildford Press, pp 409–28.

Hapak, L., Gordon, A., Locker, D., Shandling, M., Mock, D. and Tenenbaum, H.C. (1994). Differentiation between musculoligamentous, dentoalveolar, and neurologically based craniofacial pain with a diagnostic questionnaire. *Journal Orofacial Pain*, **8**: 357–68.

Woda, A., Tubert-Jeannin, S., Bouhassira, D., Attal, N., Fleiter, B., Goulet, J.P., Gremeau-Richard, C., Louise, N.M., Picard, P., Pionchon, P. *et al.* (2005). Towards a new taxonomy of idiopathic orofacial pain. *Pain*, **116**: 396–406.

Chapter 5

Overall management of facial pain

Raymond Dionne, Toby Newton-John, and Joanna M. Zakrzewska

Key points

- Most drugs used for chronic orofacial pain have not been validated in controlled clinical trials for this indication
- Limited evidence from clinical trials supports the efficacy of NSAIDs, benzodiazepines, muscle relaxants, antidepressants and anticonvulsants for the treatment of chronic orofacial pain
- No reliable evidence supports the use of corticosteroids for chronic orofacial pain
- Opioids are effective for virtually all forms of pain but should only be considered when all other treatments have failed
- Evidence based recommendations for pharmacological treatment of neuropathic pain are available and could be extrapolated for use in orofacial pain
- Psychological management needs to take place alongside other therapies
- The elements of psychological treatment include psychoeducation, self monitoring of pain, coping skills training, medication rationalization, planned follow-up with support
- Patients need access to high quality information if they are to share decisions about management and take control of their orofacial pain.

5.1 Chapter plan

Figure 5.1 is a plan of this chapter which covers the medical, surgical and psychological aspects of management which are generic to all forms of orofacial pain. Please see the individual chapters for more detail.

Figure 5.1 **Chapter plan**

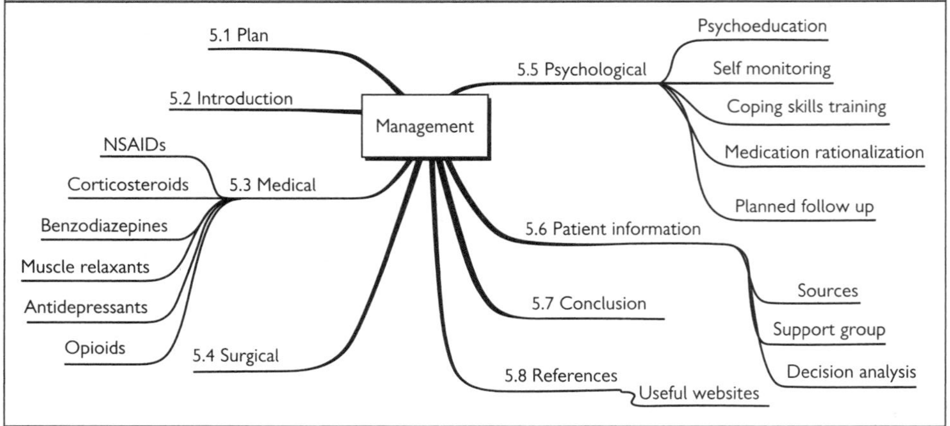

5.2 **Introduction**

In many respects treatment of a chronic facial pain patient is no different from any patient with chronic pain despite the different medical and dental causes. The same factors: gender, cultural factors, psychological influences, and genetic variation contribute to individual variation in response to painful input and so provide a rationale for individualizing pain treatment. The psychological and symbolic significance of the head in the development of self esteem, body image and interpersonal relationships, however, confers special characteristics on pain in this area.

Management should be patient centred and so requires:

- Active patient participation
- Good communication skills
- Appropriate choice of multidisciplinary treatment based on high quality evidence
- Patient information
- Encouragement of self support.

It is essential to ensure a shared understanding, achieve agreement for a treatment plan, and then ensure continued adherence. Other factors which can improve adherence to treatment are shown in Table 5.1.

This approach will:

- Ensure provision of care appropriate to patients' needs
- Improve patient safety – patients know what to expect from their treatment, check their own notes and results
- Reduce complaints and litigation – informed consent, improved communications
- Improve quality of care – patient centred satisfaction surveys and increased public accountability.

Table 5.1 Factors which improve compliance with treatments

- Provision of clear information on the origins of the pain and why it persists
- Encouraging patients to take notes during the consultation
- Providing the reasoning behind the proposed management
- Promoting positive attitude towards treatment
- Modifying schedules to suit the patients lifestyle, finances
- Providing practical solutions to how treatment can be optimized
- Encouraging patients to take on responsibility for managing their pain
- Addressing behavioural aspects of pain management
- Involving close family members in management
- Providing treatment in the context of the patients' family and culture
- Providing clear guidelines on length of treatment and goals
- Giving patient feedback and noticing their accomplishments
- Keeping information as short and simple as possible
- Regular follow up appointments with user friendly reminders if failed to attend

5.3 Medical management of facial pain

Challenges facing clinicians managing patients with orofacial pain include:

• Few clinical trials meet minimal criteria for scientific quality

• Patients' expectations of treatment now for their pain, not when an evidentiary basis exists

• Use of medications that carry significant risk with chronic administration, e.g. NSAIDs

• Use of recommendations for therapeutic decisions often extrapolated from other indications, e.g. recommendations for neuropathic pain

• Lack of appreciation of the differences between clinical observations and the need to verify the safety and effectiveness of treatments in studies that control for factors that can mimic clinical success

• History of therapeutic misadventures and a lack of scientific documentation for most clinical practices where claims of efficacy based on clinical observations are often superseded by equivocal findings of efficacy or belated recognition of adverse effects and toxicity with long-term administration

• Wide inter-individual variation in response to treatments.

The following section will provide some generic details on the major classes of drugs used in orofacial pain management with more specific information being provided in the individual chapters and in the appendix which provides lists of drug names and suggested dosages. Before prescribing any drug please check your local prescribing regulations, e.g. for the UK the British National Formulary, for the US instructions in packaged inserts, and ensure you have checked all the details as shown in Figure 2.4 (Chapter 2). Some of the commercial names for commonly used drugs are to be found in the appendix in Table 14.2.

Some simple definitions of evidence based practise are to be found in the appendix in Table 14.1. Responders to treatment are defined as those who achieved a 50% reduction in pain which in many instances is not complete pain relief.

5.3.1 NSAIDs, selective COX-2 inhibitors

While the texts and expert opinion provide recommendations for the use of NSAIDs for chronic orofacial pain, the results of placebo-controlled studies suggest that they are modestly effective for this indication. A randomized controlled trial suggests that dual COX-1 and COX-2 inhibition is needed for the treatment of orofacial pain. Selective COX-2 inhibitors such as celecoxib, however, should be considered as an alternative to NSAIDs and are likely to be better tolerated if administered chronically. Other analgesics are used for migraines and tension headaches and these are discussed in Chapter 11.

5.3.2 Topical analgesics

Topical application of an analgesic is appealing to patients and can be useful if the pain is peripheral in origin. Lidocaine injections are only practical in severe trigeminal neuralgia patients who have an identifiable trigger area and for whom a few hours relief would be beneficial. Marcaine could also be used as it is longer acting. Lidocaine patches can be used for postherpetic neuralgia and other trigeminal neuropathic pain. Intraorally small splints can be made to apply the medication but there is no high quality evidence for their use. Capsaicin cream is used in post herpetic neuralgia but it causes local side effects and so is often not well tolerated.

5.3.3 Corticosteroids

Corticosteroids are applied topically and have been injected into the TMJ in attempts to reduce the pain and dysfunction associated with chronic orofacial pain based on the hypothesis that higher drug levels can be achieved at the site of injury. One study compared dexamethasone in a lidocaine vehicle with saline placebo administered by iontophoresis three times for 5 days. Both groups of subjects (active drug and placebo) showed improvement over the course of therapy and continued to report less pain and improved range of motion at 7 and 14-day follow-ups, but did not differ from each other. This finding illustrates the dichotomy that often exists between clinical observations and the results of a clinical trial. While it appears logical to conclude that the improvement in symptoms from pre- to post-treatment was the result of the drug administered, the presence of the placebo control leads to the opposite conclusion, i.e. that the drug has no detectable benefit. In the absence of any other data, the use of steroids for chronic orofacial pain should be reserved for cases of acute trauma, severe limitation of opening or as a brief therapeutic trial. Steroids are essential in management of giant cell arteritis and this is discussed in Chapter 11.

5.3.4 Benzodiazepines

Benzodiazepines are often administered to patients with chronic pain, despite concern over their abuse potential, dependence liability and possibility of initiating or exacerbating depression. One study evaluating diazepam in comparison to placebo, demonstrated a significant decrease in orofacial pain that was attributable to diazepam. Other studies demonstrated that clonazepam was superior to placebo for burning mouth syndrome even when used topically. A study of alprazolam in fibromyalgia patients compared to placebo also showed efficacy for this chronic musculoskeletal pain conditions. Not only was the alprazolam well tolerated, some patients tapered their daily dose, contrary to a pattern of drug abuse. The results of these studies provide equivocal evidence that benzodiazepines provide relief from musculoskeletal orofacial pain. Conversely, benzodiazepines should not be prescribed in large amounts that would permit dose escalation. Lack of treatment response or over-sedation should prompt a reduction in dose or discontinuation. Therapy with a benzodiazepine should not be continued beyond a few weeks and lack of a therapeutic response should prompt re-evaluation rather than an increased dose or long-term treatment.

5.3.5 **Muscle relaxants**

Drugs that reduce muscle tension are often administered in an attempt to relax increased muscle activity associated with orofacial pain of muscular origin. Muscle relaxant drugs are thought to decrease muscle tone by acting centrally to depress polysynaptic reflexes. Drugs with sedative properties, e.g. benzodiazepines also reduce muscle tone and are used for orofacial pain of presumed muscular origin in part due to their putative muscle relaxant properties. Of the drugs available for clinical use, cyclobenzaprine has been demonstrated to be superior to placebo in clinical trials for pain in cervical and lumbar regions associated with skeletal muscle spasms and reduces electro-myographic signs of muscle spasm. While little evidence exists for the efficacy of muscle relaxants for orofacial pain, use of muscle relaxants for increased muscle tone associated with orofacial pain including chronic tension headaches may be useful for a brief trial in conjunction with physical therapy.

5.3.6 **Antidepressants**

Antidepressants have been used in the treatment of pain for approximately 30 years, including orofacial pain. The two main groups are the older tricyclic ·antidepressants such as amitriptyline, dosulepin and the newer selective serotonin re-uptake inhibitors (SSRI) such as fluoxetine, or serotonin noradrenaline re-uptake inhibitors (SNRI) such as venlafaxine or duloxetine. Critical appraisal of their analgesic and antidepressant activities indicates that the analgesic effect of this drug class is largely independent of antidepressant activity. Further details can be found in the Neuropathic Pain volume in the series (Chapter 9). Analgesia can be differentiated from placebo effects, occurs at doses lower that those used for depression and are demonstrated in non-depressed patients. Studies of neuropathic pain indicate that drugs that inhibit reuptake of both serotonin and noradrenaline are more efficacious than drugs that are selective for either of these neurotransmitters. For neuropathic pain recent guidelines have suggested the use of duloxetine or venlafaxine. One study in patients with chronic orofacial pain demonstrated that amitriptyline in a daily dose of approximately 25 mg was equally effective as higher doses (>100 mg). A dose-response comparison of 25, 50 and 75 mg of amitriptyline is reported to result in increased analgesia with increasing dose and improved sleep for the 75 mg dose but with significantly higher incidence of adverse effects for this dose. Recent guidelines on neuropathic pain management suggest the use of nortriptyline up to maximum of 150 mg in preference to amitriptyline. In general doses lower than those used in depression are used for pain.

For patients who are mildly depressed or have a sleep disorder, low doses of tricyclic antidepressants may be considered. A recent systematic review of SSRIs suggests these drugs are only effective in patients with major depression.

5.3.7 **Anticonvulsants/anti-epileptics**

This class of drug is mainly used in the management of trigeminal neuralgia and will be discussed in detail in Chapter 10. The newer ones such as gabapentin and pregabalin act on a variety of receptors including α2 δ calcium channel ligands and it is this structural difference that makes them effective in neuropathic pain and even TMD. The doses used are similar to those used in epilepsy. Adverse side effects are similar in all these drugs which include drowsiness, ataxia and fatigue.

5.3.8 **Opioids**

Use of opioids for non-malignant pain is controversial but should be considered for orofacial pain under some circumstances. A large body of research demonstrates that orally administered opioids result in significant analgesia without respiratory depression, but with an increased incidence of adverse effects in comparison with placebo or non-opioid drugs. Most concern over the use of opioids for chronic pain relates to their potential for 'addiction'.

Opioids should be considered when:
- More conservative measures have failed
- Patient may be at risk for the serious adverse effects associated with chronic NSAID administration
- Additional TMJ surgery is being contemplated that might produce iatrogenic injury
- Neuropathic pain which has failed to respond to other drugs.
- Prescribing a sustained-release formulation should minimize cyclic fluctuations in pain associated with standard formulations with a short duration of action.

Chronic administration of opioids requires careful:
- Patient selection to rule out drug-seeking behaviour
- Monitoring to individualize the dose and minimize side effects
- Attention to regulatory procedures.

With patients for whom other therapeutic modalities have failed, or another therapeutic approach is not readily apparent, a trial with an opioid should be considered. Although tolerance and dependence need to be considered, opioids may represent a more favourable therapeutic alternative than risk of iatrogenic injury from further surgeries or experimentation with non-validated clinical practices.

5.3.9 **Triptans**

This class of drug is highly specific for migraine type pain and is further discussed in Chapters 11 and 12.

5.3.10 **Therapeutic Recommendations**

Due to lack of evidence-based practice in this area; clinicians should be cognizant that use of some drug classes are non-validated clinical practices and limit treatment to short trials to evaluate clinical efficacy and potential adverse effects. Figure 5.2 provides some indication for use of various drug classes.

Figure 5.2 Major groups of drugs used in orofacial pain

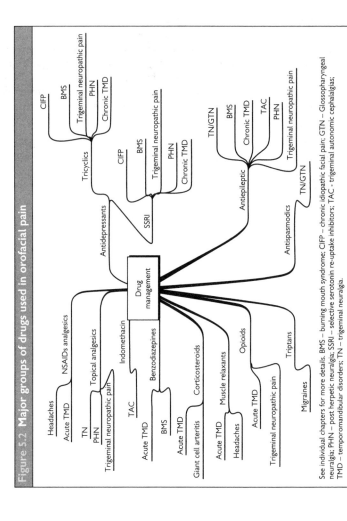

See individual chapters for more details. BMS – burning mouth syndrome; CIFP – chronic idiopathic facial pain; GTN – Glossopharyngeal neuralgia; PHN – post herpetic neuralgia; SSRI – selective serotonin re-uptake inhibitors; TAC - trigeminal autonomic cephalalgias; TMD – temporomandibular disorders; TN – trigeminal neuralgia.

5.4 **Surgical management of facial pain**

There are very few surgical procedures that are used in the management of facial pain with the exception of trigeminal neuralgia. Selective nerve destruction, decompression of nerves, arthrocentesis, arthroscopy, TMJ disc repositioning, menisectomy, TMJ reconstruction are some that are in use but as they are irreversible procedures they should be avoided if there is no clear indication for their use.

Dental treatment should only be carried out when there is a clinical indication and these are covered in Chapter 6.

5.5 **Psychological management**

The primary objective of psychological treatment for chronic orofacial pain is to reduce or minimize the suffering that accompanies the experience of intractable pain. There are times when recourse to specialist clinical psychology input is necessary, however all clinicians can promote the following skills when dealing with their patients, in order to maximize good coping and a sense of resilience. This is summarized in Figure 5.3.

5.5.1 **Psychoeducation**

To begin with, patients with persistent orofacial pain problems require good quality information about their condition. Pain normally indicates a threat to the organism; threat creates fear, and fear in turn can exacerbate the experience of pain. Reducing the sense of threat begins with better knowledge of the pain itself. Busy clinicians should arm themselves with 'bibliotherapy' resources that they are familiar with and trust. Better still, clinicians can develop their own written materials relating to the conditions that are most commonly seen in the clinic. That way, the clinician can ensure that he or she can give out written information (remember, the vast majority of what is discussed in a consultation is forgotten quickly afterwards) which addresses the issues that their patient population is most likely to have. A list of web-based information sites is given after this chapter to help guide the reading and an example of a leaflet provided in the appendix.

Part of the psychoeducational component of treatment should include information about the nature of chronic pain itself. Many patients will be extremely defensive about discussing their emotional state, due to anxieties that an expression of distress might lead to their pain being an interpreted as a psychological problem rather than a 'real', physical one. Having outlined the known or presumed biological components of the pain problem, the clinician can then introduce the chronic pain model in which biopsychosocial factors are all relevant to the pain experience.

Figure 5.3 Psychological management of facial pain

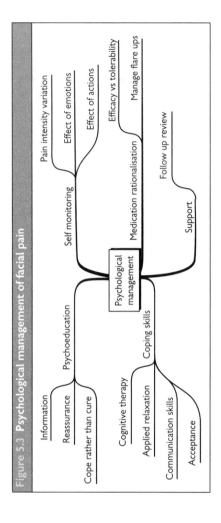

The chronic pain model also emphasises the intractable nature of pain once phenomena such as central and peripheral sensitisation, 'wind up' and cortical reorganization have become established. As part of the psychoeducational aspect of the intervention, helping patients to understand that the treatment goal is often management of the pain rather than its complete elimination is important. The desire to be free of pain is an understandably strong one, yet patient suffering can be reduced when expectations are brought more into line with reality. The notion of acceptance of pain is discussed further below.

5.5.2 **Self-monitoring**

Many orofacial pain patients find it difficult to identify the precipitants of variation in their pain levels. It can be helpful then for patients to monitor their pain levels over the course of several weeks in order to better understand what factors are associated with episodes of increased pain as well as decreased pain. A simple exercise as shown in Table 5.2 is to ask patients to rate their pain experience in three domains at the end of each day: their average pain level (0–10 numerical rating scale); when their pain was at its best (rated 0–10, plus what they were doing at the time and what they were thinking at the time); and when it was at its worst (with similar 0–10 rating as well as their thoughts and actions at the time).

By tracking the pain like this for a short period, patients can begin to see patterns developing which they may be unaware of, such as pain worsening after spousal disagreements or improving on the weekends when stress levels are lower.

One caveat to this sort of self-monitoring exercise is to keep it time limited. Focusing on pain is useful in order to better understand its antecedents and consequences, but the clinician must be careful that this exercise does not increase negative rumination on the pain or increase anxiety in the more obsessional patient. A two to three week monitoring period will provide more than enough relevant information without creating a new 'hobby' of charting every movement of the pain.

5.5.3 **Coping skills training**

The management of persistent pain is a question of how individuals respond to their pain – what they do, or don't do, as a reaction to their sensory experience. The cognitive therapy model is based on the simple premise that

63

Table 5.2 **Example of self monitoring diary of pain**					
Date	**Over course of day score pain from 0–10: 0 = no pain, 10 = worse pain**				
	Lowest score	Actions feelings	Highest score	Actions feelings	Average score
6th June	3	Playing with grandchildren Happy	7	In a traffic jam Angry, frustrated	5

thoughts or cognitions directly impact upon the emotional state, and the combination of cognition and emotion then determines the behavioural response to a given situation.

The notion of 'catastrophizing' refers to a thinking style in which pain is interpreted in its most negative and alarmist fashion, e.g.

• 'This pain is overwhelming'
• 'There is nothing I can do to control the pain'
• 'This flare up will never go away'.

Catastrophic thinking leads to:

• Catastrophic emotions, such as fear, anxiety and extreme stress
• Maladaptive responses to pain such as excessive medication taking
• Helplessness
• Further treatment seeking.

5.5.3.1 *Thought challenging*

Helping chronic pain patients to identify their pain cognitions (most recognize the emotional consequences of pain but find that deciphering the self-talk that results in those emotions is more difficult) is an important aspect of pain coping skills training. It is also the first step in developing the technique of 'thought challenging', a cognitive therapy method in which the maladaptive thinking is replaced by more rational, logical or helpful interpretations of the given situation.

5.5.3.2 *Applied relaxation techniques*

Complementary to cognitive techniques such as thought challenging are the arousal reduction techniques such as applied relaxation skills. Patients who become highly distressed by their pain often derive benefit from being shown simple, rapidly effective breathing or imagery techniques which decrease their stress levels. It is important that patients understand that such methods are designed to reduce arousal levels (e.g. muscle tension, heart rate, blood pressure) rather than decrease the pain itself. It is also important that such techniques are portable and self-directed, so that the patient can initiate a stress-reduction response when and wherever he or she happens to be when the pain builds. This is particularly important for trigeminal neuralgia sufferers, whose experience of 'attacks' may come on suddenly and with little preparatory time.

5.5.3.3 *Communication skills*

Teaching patients how to communicate effectively with others regarding their pain is often an overlooked element of coping skills training. The majority of pain patients will say that they dislike talking about their pain, and keep their discussions of pain to a minimum. Yet these same patients are also the ones whose non-verbal pain behaviour, such as grimacing, eye rolling, medication taking and resting, is often extremely overt. Hence there are often mixed messages being sent, which can cause confusion and resentment in partners and close family members who are potential sources of support. Chronic pain patients need to

- Communicate clearly and concisely about their pain
- Decrease their displays of pain behaviour
- Reduce negative feelings in others.

Formal couples counselling or marital therapy may become necessary if the resentments about the pain have become pronounced.

5.5.3.4 *Acceptance*

Recently psychologists have suggested adopting a less control-seeking approach to pain management (such as with cognitive restructuring exercises) and instead pursuing more of an acceptance-based or mindfulness approach to the pain. Stemming from an Eastern philosophical perspective, acceptance-based therapies for chronic pain take the view that patient efforts to escape pain, such as by taking medications, resting and 'doctor shopping', are often more debilitating than the pain itself. By helping patients to accept their pain – to stop struggling to escape from the inescapable – more energy is left to devote to pursuing valued life goals, the identification of which is also an important element of treatment.

5.5.4 **Medication rationalization**

Many chronic orofacial pain patients accumulate pain medications as they move around the healthcare system from doctor to dentist to specialist and back again. Often doses escalate without any corresponding improvement in pain or functional activity level, yet the side effect profile continues to grow and can cause more interference in day to day life than the pain itself. It is essential to explore gradual weaning down on medications as the reduction in side effects may more than compensate for any minor change in pain intensity. It is particularly important that while medication is gradually being withdrawn, the patient is shown alternative methods for responding to the pain such as those listed above. This includes specific strategies for dealing with pain flares.

5.5.5 **Planned follow up and support**

Living with chronic pain is a challenge, and requires significant psychological strength and resilience. Having a planned follow up period after the conclusion of the intervention is important for the patient in knowing that support is ongoing. There will undoubtedly be times where the patient does not manage well and the flare up becomes overwhelming, but having that support in place is both reassuring and containing. Again, enlisting the significant other in providing that support for the long term can be a valuable investment

5.6 **Patient information and decision making**

Patient centred care requires patients to have access to good quality information. This has led to pilot schemes in the UK called 'Information Prescriptions' which work like a sign posting service – providing patients with the right information, at the right time. Patients are presented with a range of information and choose those sections that are of interest to them personally. These are then 'stored' on the internet for current or later use. The information can be provided in many formats:

- Leaflets
- Books
- Videos
- Internet
- Support groups.

However, like all treatments quality control is essential and care must be taken when selecting information and the clinician can help in this as detailed in section 5.5.1. Organizations like DISCERN, or Centre for Health Information Quality provide tools to judge the quality of information on the internet.

5.6.1 **Self help/support groups**

Long term conditions such as chronic orofacial pain require patients to take control of their condition and they can be helped to do this through patient groups. Some of these are listed at the end of the chapter.

Self help groups aim to

- Decrease patients' sense of isolation
- Show that there are others who care
- Provide new ways of coping
- Provide a forum for sharing feelings
- Increase confidence in asking questions from healthcare providers.

Support groups have a slightly different remit in that they also aim to

- Provide information about the disease/condition
- Increase public and professional awareness of the condition
- Put patients in touch with each other
- Look for available resources for treatment.

5.6.2 **Decision making**

Making decisions about treatment depends not only on the patients' understanding of the condition but also their understanding and attitude towards risk taking. Risk taking involves assessing the probability, severity and timing of an adverse outcome as well as the positive outcome. Some patients will want the healthcare professionals to make the decisions for them; others will wish to share this task with their healthcare professional whereas others will want to make the decisions on their own. This process takes time and patience is needed by the health care professionals when working with pain patients. See Table 5.3.

Table 5.3 Elements involved in shared decision making

For shared decision-making (SDM) four steps must take place:

1. Both the patient and the doctor need to be involved

2. Both parties share information

3. Both parties take steps to build a consensus about the preferred treatment

4. An agreement is reached on the treatment to implement

SDM improves informed consent and leads to improved health outcomes

In order to take part in SDM, patients must

- Be fully informed of all the options available and this will involve accessing medical literature, web sites and patient information data

- Understand the pros and cons of all the procedures, including the tradeoffs and be able to interpret the data including the assessment of risk

- Take into account their own beliefs

Most pain patients will have multiple complaints which will sometimes include depression, and so a single modality approach is unlikely to work. This may not only involve the use of several different methods but also an interdisciplinary team of healthcare workers.

5.7 **Conclusions**

Management of orofacial pain requires a biopsychosocial approach in which physical therapies, drugs, potentially surgery, psychological techniques are all used alongside each other in order to enable patients to gain enough information to self manage their pain.

5.8 **References**

Bennett, M. (2006). *Neuropathic Pain,* Oxford University Press, Oxford.

Cole, F., Macdonald, H., Carus, C., Howden-Leach, H. (2005). *Overcoming Chronic pain,* Robinson, London.

Dellemijn, P.L., Fields, H.L. (1994). Do benzodiazepines have a role in chronic pain management? *Pain,* **57**: 137–52.

Dionne, R.A., Kim, H., Gordon, S.M. (2006). Acute and chronic dental and orofacial pain. In (eds) McMahon, S.B., Koltzenburg, M., *Wall and Melzack's Textbook of Pain,* pp 819–35. Elsevier, Philadelphia.

Feinmann, C. (1999). *The Mouth, the Face and the Mind.* Oxford University Press, Oxford.

List, T., Axelson, S., Leijon, G. (2003). Pharmacological interventions in the treatment of temporomandibular disorders, atypical facial pain, and burning mouth syndrome: A qualitative systematic review. *Journal Orofacial Pain,* **17**: 301–10.

Lund, J.P., Lavigne, G.J., Dubner, R. and Sessle, B.J. (2001). *Orofacial Pain, from Basic Science to Clinical Management.* Quintessence Publishing Co.Inc, Chicago.

Lee, J., Baranowski, A. (2007). *Long-term Pain – a guide to practical management,* Oxford University Press, Oxford.

Muir Gray, J.A., Rutter, H. (2002). *The Resourceful Patient.* eRosetta Press, Oxford. This is also a Web based book. http://www.resourcefulpatient.org/

Newton-John, T. (2002). Psychology of pain. In: Zakrzewska, J. and Harrison, S. (eds) *Assessment and Management of Orofacial Pain,* Volume 14. pp 35–52. Elsevier Press, Amsterdam.

Paling, J. (2003). Strategies to help patients understand risks. *British Medical Journal,* **327**: 745–48.

Useful websites

American Pain Foundation http://www.painfoundation.org/

Bandolier, The Oxford Pain Internet Site http://www.medicine.ox.ac.uk/Bandolier/booth/painpag/index2.html

British Pain Society http://www.britishpainsociety.org/

Cluster headaches resources http://www.chhelp.org, http://www.clusterheadaches.org/

DISCERN http://www.discern.org.uk/

The Expert Patient Programme http://www.dh.gov.uk/en/Publicationsandstatistics/Publications/PublicationsPolicyAndGuidance/DH_4006801

International Association for the Study of Pain http://www.iasp-pain.org

National Guideline Clearing House http://www.guideline.gov

Neuropathy Trust http://www.neurocentre.com

Patient Decision-making/Patient Choice Initiative http://www.kingsfund.org.uk/library

The TMJ Association http://www.tmj.org/

US trigeminal neuralgia http://www.tna-support.org

UK trigeminal neuralgia http://www.tna-uk.org.uk

Chapter 6

Dental causes of orofacial pain

Edward R. Vickers and Joanna M. Zakrzewska

> **Key points**
> - Dental causes of orofacial pain are common in the population
> - Different pain qualities exist in the stages of dental pulpitis
> - Dental causes of pain can be identified through detailed clinical examination and radiographs
> - Co-existing dental pathologies are important to identify
> - Acute and chronic pain states may be concurrent
> - Maxillary sinusitis has several diagnostic features that enable rapid diagnosis without the need for imaging
> - Salivary gland diseases can present without chronic pain

6.1 Chapter plan

Figure 6.1 is an outline of the main contents of the chapter.

6.2 Introduction

Dental and oral disease states are recognized as the most common pathology to afflict the general population. Dental disease such as caries is the primary cause of patients seeking pain relief from dental practitioners. However, acute dental pain in the trigeminal nerve distribution can be the possible result of numerous and potentially concurrent causative factors. Anatomically these factors can be broadly classified into diseases affecting

1. teeth (i.e. typically dental carious lesions and subsequent stimulation of the dental pulp)
2. adjacent soft tissues of gingivae and oral mucosa (dental abscess and oral ulceration)
3. bone and orofacial pathology (e.g. jaw fracture and infection such as osteomyelitis)

Figure 6.1 Chapter plan

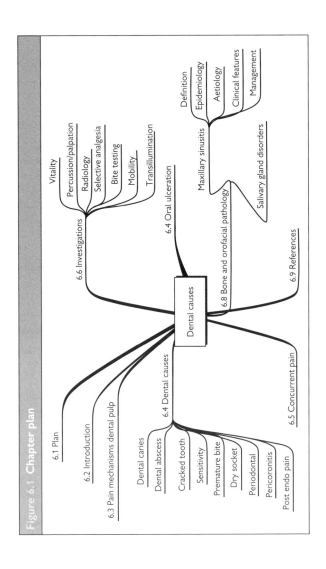

6.3 **Pain mechanisms of the dental pulp**

There are two clinical descriptions of pulpal pain. These are mediated by different nerve fibres.

One clinical pain description is of a short, sharp, brief pain that is induced by the rapid fluid flow within dentinal tubules from stimuli such as cold, heat, air, drilling and osmotic changes. Typically this pain is the physiological 'helpful' warning response in order to prevent ongoing noxious stimuli damaging the pulp.

The second clinical description is reported as a slow, dull, aching, poorly localized pain indicating the presence of inflammatory mediators on nerve fibres and established pulpal inflammation. Pain of this type often requires extirpation (removal) of the pulp or tooth extraction to relieve the patient from his/her pain, i.e. the Cartesian 'amputation' approach to pain relief.

There are progressive stages of pain from the physiological (reversible) pain to the second (irreversible) pain necessitating endodontic treatment or tooth extraction:

1. Brief, sharp pain from thermal stimulation that resolves immediately after removal of the stimulus
2. Brief, sharp pain followed by prolonged, dull ache that eventually dissipates (potentially reversible pulpitis)
3. Increased pain intensity to noxious stimuli and dull ache that is constant or recurrent over days and weeks (potentially irreversible pulpitis)
4. Constant, severe, unrelenting toothache (acute pulpitis)
5. No pain response to noxious stimulus (non-vital tooth)
6. Periapical infection in bone and tenderness and pain to percussion.

There is usually minor pain where adequate discharge of pus is occurring from a sinus tract, or severe pain where there is little drainage present.

Identification of the exact tooth in the early stages is best carried out with cold water spray under rubber dam.

6.4 **Specific causes of dental pain**

6.4.1 **Dental caries**

Carious lesions occur in enamel, dentine and cementum. Enamel is avascular and nonporous. Demineralization of enamel occurs without pain. Once the carious lesion has broached the enamel-dentine interface then pain may be noticed from stimuli affecting the dentinal tubules. Caries may also occur on exposed root surfaces where cementum overlying dentine is thin. Caries can proceed very rapidly in special patient groups where xerostomia is present from radiation oncology treatment for head and neck cancer. Treatment of caries is removal of decay and placement of a dental restoration. Prevention of caries utilizes optimum dental hygiene techniques of brushing, flossing and fluoride applications. Figure 6.2 shows caries.

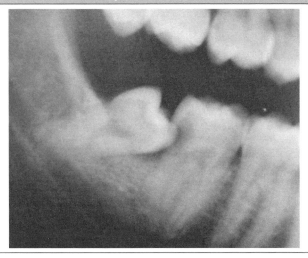

Figure 6.2 **Dental radiographic pathologies of caries on the distal aspect of 2nd molar and impacted 3rd molar**

6.4.2 **Dental abscess**

Dental periapical abscess is the subsequent result of caries and irreversible pulpitis. Other causes may be trauma to the teeth or spread of infection from distant sites via blood supply into the pulp (rare). In addition, infection can occur in the lateral aspect of the tooth from root fracture or infection (lateral periodontal abscess). Drainage of infection, antibiotics and dental treatment (extraction or endodontics) are the treatment principles.

6.4.3 **Cracked teeth syndrome**

Patients with bruxism (tooth grinding and jaw clenching) can exert tremendous degrees of force on the teeth. Enamel is hard and brittle that results in cracks. Occasionally these cracks can extend through the enamel and into the dentine causing pain. Dental treatment involves removal of the crack and appropriate restorative measures depending on the extent of the crack. In addition, occlusal splints can be fabricated to reduce loading forces on affected teeth and instituting psychological techniques such as relaxation training where background stress is a causative factor in bruxism.

6.4.4 **Sensitivity from dental restorations**

Pain can result from dental restorations in several ways:

- Composite resin restorations may not provide adequate barrier protection against thermal stimuli.
- An inadequate lining material between the restoration such as a large metal restoration in close proximity to the dental pulp

- Dental restorations may expand and break the tooth-restoration seal resulting in 'leaking' and pain from a fluid stimulus such as cold water
- Galvanic effects occur where metallic restorations contact each other to set up a galvanic cell through the ionic nature of saliva. Although infrequently used in current dentistry a newly placed amalgam restoration contacting an old amalgam or gold restoration can result in a 'tingling' pain sensation.

Treatment is replacement or use of alternative dental materials.

6.4.5 **Exposed cementum or dentine**

The tooth root surface (a thin layer of cementum overlaying dentine) is exposed from excessive or incorrect tooth brushing. There is tooth sensitivity from cold fluids/air and treatment includes restorations, applications of desensitizing agents and correction of tooth brushing technique.

6.4.6 **Premature contact ('high bite')**

This is characterized by a sharp pain (then a dull ache if problem persists) due to a recent tooth restoration that is 'high' compared with the normal occlusion when biting together. Identification and reduction of the premature contact resolves the pain.

6.4.7 **Alveolar osteitis ('dry socket')**

Usually occurs 1–3 days after a tooth extraction when the blood clot in the socket is lost through mechanical means (excessive and vigorous rinsing), smoking or possible fibrinolytic substances in saliva. Patients complain of a deep, aching, radiating pain originating in the extraction site from exposed nerve endings in the wall of the socket. Pain is only partially relieved by typical dental analgesics (codeine/ paracetamol/ibuprofen). Treatment involves local topical application of medicaments to chemically cauterize exposed nerve endings and more potent analgesics and sedatives for breakthrough pain.

6.4.8 **Gingivitis and periodontitis**

Gingivitis (bleeding gums) is usually painless while periodontitis may exhibit an episodic, low intensity, dull pain due to inflammation and infection. Where infection is present treatment requires antibiotics with follow up periodontal treatment and meticulous oral hygiene.

6.4.9 **Pericoronitis**

Infected tissue usually associated with an impacted or erupting lower third molar (wisdom) tooth. Antibiotics for the acute infection and analgesics for pain relief with surgical removal of the impacted tooth are treatment principles.

6.4.10 **Post endodontic surgery pain**

Severe, aching pain following endodontic treatment (root canal therapy or apicectomy). While the majority of patients improve over time (weeks), a patient can develop neurogenic inflammation and neuropathic pain. Further detail is provided in Chapter 11, Section 11.2.

6.5 **Co-existing (concurrent) trigeminal pain states and referred pain**

It is important to recognize that acute pain can co-exist at times with chronic pain. Different pains require assessment, detection and knowledge of acute and chronic pain.

- There may be separate co-existing pain states in the trigeminal nerve, e.g. acute pulpitis in a tooth and an attack of trigeminal neuralgia. Similarly, cracked tooth syndrome from bruxism with concurrent myofascial pain in the jaw closing muscles
- Acute dental pulpitis can refer pain to a non-decayed tooth in a same or ipsilateral quadrant
- Body pain can refer to the orofacial region, e.g. angina can refer pain to the left mandible, maxillary sinusitis can refer pain to the maxillary teeth.

6.6 **Investigations for dental pathology**

6.6.1 **Vitality tests**

Vitality tests employ hot, cold and electrical testing stimuli. The test should be conducted by isolating and testing teeth on an individual basis and comparison testing of a number of adjacent teeth. Results to identify a painful tooth can be variable and are more useful for exclusion of normal responsive teeth. Pulp testing is helpful if all teeth are responding normally suggesting pain is from a non-dental cause, or identifying the non-responsive causative tooth where there is an obvious dental infection.

6.6.2 **Percussion**

Percussion is useful for determining the individual painful tooth but caution should be used where numerous teeth are painful to percussion as this may indicate widespread infection or bruxism.

6.6.3 **Palpation**

Palpation of adjacent supporting bone can indicate swelling associated with an infected tooth.

6.6.4 **Radiographs**

Radiographs are a standard technique for assessing dental health and pathology. Intraoral radiographs are ideal for dental caries and periapical lesions. In cases of irreversible pulpitis the corresponding changes in bone architecture may not be visible for two weeks and a repeat radiograph is necessary. A dental panoramic radiograph is an excellent first line radiograph to view potential pathology of the maxilla, mandible, sinuses and temporomandibular joints. Further detail is provided in Chapter 3, Section 3.3.

6.6.5 Selective anaesthesia

Selective anaesthesia is useful for identifying pain from a branch of the trigeminal nerve in areas of possible referred pain. Caution should be used when identifying the exact painful tooth from selective anaesthesia. For example, due to the spread of the local anaesthetic a false positive reading may result in a suspected diseased tooth that is actually healthy. Correspondingly, there is a false negative reading to the unknown adjacent diseased tooth.

6.6.6 Bite testing

Bite testing is distinguishable from percussion particularly on cracked teeth. Percussion to a cracked tooth is only evident when the force is in the direction that opens the crack. Lateral jaw excursions with teeth contacting each other are more likely to yield the source of the pain.

6.6.7 Mobility

A mobile tooth due to infection is clearly distinguishable from adjacent healthy teeth. Where multiple, non-painful, mobile teeth are present the likely diagnosis is periodontal disease.

6.6.8 Transillumination

This technique is helpful for visualizing cracks in teeth, particularly vertical cracks (bruxism) and oblique cracks in corners of restorations and cavity preparations.

6.7 Oral ulceration

An ulcer is defined as a breach in the epithelium that exposes the underlying connective tissue. In the oral cavity tissues are enriched with nerve fibres and nociception occurs from numerous stimuli. Oral ulceration in the majority of cases is self limiting, e.g. traumatic ulcer. However, several systemic medical conditions exhibit recurrent pan-oral ulceration. It can be painful, socially distressing and discomfort from eating compromises bodily nutritional needs.

The aetiology of oral ulceration is varied and can be broadly grouped as traumatic (mechanical, thermal, chemical), infection, autoimmune, hormonal (pregnancy/oestrus cycle), nutritional deficiency (iron, vitamin B_{12}, folate), food intolerance/sensitivity, psychological stress, and as a drug-induced side effect. The classification of oral ulceration is dependent on the aetiology, if known and Table 6.1 shows a detailed list with the more common ones highlighted. Non-healing ulcers warrant biopsy to exclude squamous cell carcinoma. The treatment for oral ulceration largely utilizes topical agents containing a mixture of local anaesthetic agents, anti-inflammatory agents, astringents and antibacterial agents. In autoimmune diseases steroids are usually administered for medical reasons with an improvement in oral discomfort.

As there is a lesion to see as well as pain it is not often that these are mistaken for other types of pain discussed in this book.

Table 6.1 Types of oral ulceration causing oral pain

Traumatic
(a) Morsicatio buccarum (cheek biting)*
(b) Other traumatic self induced (lip, tongue, hot food etc)
(c) Cotton roll ulcer
(d) Factitial ulcer

Iatrogenic
(a) Traumatic (self, surgical instrument)
(b) Aspirin burn
(c) Contact stomatitis (amalgam allergy)
(d) Radiation mucositis
(e) Lichenoid drug reaction (gold, antihypertensives)

Idiopathic
(a) Aphthous – minor *, major, herpetiform

Autoimmune
(a) Behçet's syndrome
(b) Erythema migrans *
(c) Lupus erythematosus (discoid and systemic)
(d) Pemphigus vulgaris
(e) Mucous membrane pemphigoid
(f) Lichen planus *
(g) Erythema multiforme
(h) Crohn's disease

Infection (local and systemic)
(a) Primary herpetic gingivostomatitis *
(b) Recurrent herpes stomatitis *
(c) Chronic herpes simplex
(d) Herpes zoster
(e) Herpangina
(f) Tuberculosis
(g) Syphilitic chancre, gumma
(h) Histoplasmosis, blastomycosis
(i) Hand, foot and mouth disease

* More common conditions.

6.8 Bone and orofacial pathology

Bone pathology causing pain in the trigeminal nerve encompasses a wide range of cysts, benign tumours, malignancy, infection and facial trauma. See Figure 6.3 showing a large cyst.

In addition specific pain states such as avascular osteonecrosis are becoming more common.

6.8.1 Maxillary sinusitis

6.8.1.1 Definition

This is defined as a 'constant burning pain with zygomatic and dental tenderness from the inflammation of the maxillary sinus'. Most sinusitis is acute

Figure 6.3 Pain caused by dental pathology of an infected cyst associated with an impacted third molar tooth

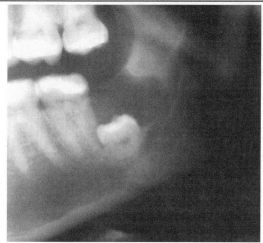

and the chronic form is less likely to be associated with pain. The International Headache Society suggests that the diagnostic criteria for all the sinusitis is the same and the only difference is the location and specific headache. These are shown below:

- Purulent discharge in the nasal passage either spontaneous or by suction
- Pathological findings in one or more of the following tests
- X-ray examination
- Computerized tomography or magnetic resonance imaging
- Transillumination
- Simultaneous onset of headache and sinusitis
- Headache location – in acute maxillary sinusitis headache is located over the antral area and may radiate to the upper teeth or the forehead
- Headache disappears after treatment of acute sinusitis.

6.8.1.2 *Epidemiology*
It is estimated that 0.5–5% of all upper respiratory tract infections will be complicated by maxillary sinusitis.

6.8.1.3 *Aetiology*
Acute sinusitis is most frequently caused by viral or bacterial causes. Viral and bacterial sinusitis are difficult to differentiate on clinical grounds. Patients with prolonged viral upper respiratory tract infection (common cold) may go on to develop sinusitis. Bacterial sinusitis tends to be present if symptoms have lasted more than 7 days. The most commonly implicated bacteria are the *Streptococcus*

pneumoniae and *Haemophilus influenzae*. It can occur after a dental infection or after treatment to upper premolar or molars especially extractions.

6.8.1.4 *Clinical features*
The clinical features are shown in Figure 6.4

It has been suggested that there is a higher likelihood of bacterial infection when the following are present:
- Maxillary tooth or facial pain (especially unilateral)
- Purulent nasal discharge
- Unilateral maxillary sinus tenderness
- Worsening of symptoms after initial improvement.

6.8.1.5 **Examination**
There will be tenderness over the affected cheek and occasionally some redness. Intra-orally the upper teeth on the affected area will be tender to percussion. The sinus can be transilluminated by putting a torch in intra-orally.

6.8.1.6 *Investigations*
Although maxillary sinus radiography and CT scanning will be positive in 90% of bacterial sinusitis they often do not add any further information to that obtained clinically.

6.8.1.7 *Management*
This should begin with symptomatic treatments; these are numerous but few have been proven to be efficacious in RCTs. The following are used:
- Decongestants
- Analgesics
- Alpha-adrenergic agents
- Mucolytic agents
- Antihistamines
- Corticosteriods
- Proteolytic agents.

The indications for antibiotic use include
- Moderately severe symptoms and acute bacterial sinusitis
- Symptoms lasting more than 7 days
- Pain of face or teeth
- Purulent nasal secretions
- Severe symptoms regardless of duration.

Expert opinion concludes that if an antibiotic is required it should be the most narrow spectrum active against the most likely pathogens of *S. pneumoniae* and *H. influenzae*. There are several Cochrane reviews of antibiotics to be used and they have shown that amoxycillin is the drug of choice.

Most patients should be well in 7–10 days but community studies have shown that up to a quarter of patients may have symptoms lasting over 13 days.

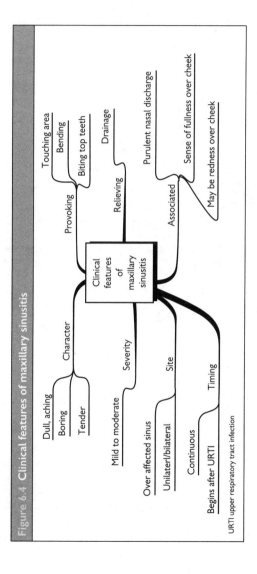

Figure 6.4 Clinical features of maxillary sinusitis

URTI upper respiratory tract infection

6.8.2 **Salivary gland pathology**

Tumours, duct blockage and subsequent infection also elicit pain in the trigeminal nerve.

Salivary stones are most frequent in the submandibular gland. The pain is intermittent and characteristically occurs just before eating. There may be associated tenderness of the involved salivary gland. Bimanual palpation will enable the stone to be palpated if it is in the duct and salivary flow from the duct will be slow or absent. The picture in Figure 6.5 shows a salivary stone being taken out using a small basket device.

More detailed information on the diagnosis and treatment of these disease and pain states can be readily sourced from specific texts.

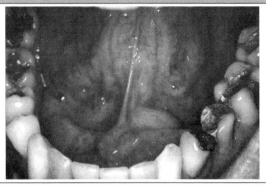

Figure 6.5 Salivary stone being removed from the submandibular duct using a basket device

Acknowledgments

We are very grateful to Professor Alex Moule, School of Dentistry, University of Queensland for providing information for this chapter.

6.9 **References**

Hargreaves, K.M., Goodis, H.E. (2002). *Seltzer and Bender's dental pulp*. Quintessence, Hanover Park, IL.

Hasselgren, G. (2000). Pains of dental origin. In: Dym, H. Ed. *Diagnosis and management of facial pain. Oral and Maxillofacial Clinics of North America*. WB Saunders, Philadephia. 12, 2, pp 263–4.

Little, J.W., Falace, D.A. (1993). *Dental management of the medically compromised patient*. 4th ed. Mosby, St Louis.

Mahan, P.E., Alling, C.C. (1991). *Facial pain*. 3rd ed. Lea and Febiger, Philadelphia.

Therapeutic Guidelines Ltd and Australian Dental Association. (2007). *Therapeutic Guidelines Oral and Dental.* Version 1. Therapeutic Guidelines Ltd, Nth Melbourne.

Vickers, E.R. (2005). *Orofacial pain: problem based learning.* Sydney University Press.

Weiner, S.L. (1993). *Differential diagnosis of acute pain by body region.* McGraw-Hill, New York.

Chapter 7

Burning mouth syndrome (BMS)

Alain Woda and Miriam Grushka

Key points
• BMS remains an enigmatic pain condition
• Pathogenesis needs to explain the multiple sensory changes that are reported
• Clinical features are distinctive with burning of the oral mucosa associated with taste disturbance and xerostomia
• Few randomized controlled trials are available to guide therapy
• Medication therapy is with low-doses of anxiolytics, antidepressants and anticonvulsant agents, both topically and systemically
• Psychological support is crucial and has been shown to be beneficial.

7.1 Chapter plan

Figure 7.1 is an outline of the main contents of this chapter.

7.2 Definition

Burning mouth syndrome (BMS) is characterized by continuous burning pain of the oral mucosa with spontaneous onset, which usually cannot be attributed to pain from local or systemic pathology. When oral burning pain is the result of a known disease process, it should be clearly distinguished from burning mouth syndrome in that the burning is a symptom which results from a specific etiology such as pharmacological treatment or local/systemic pathological conditions. It has been suggested that terms such as 'stomatodynia' be used only to refer to primary burning mouth syndrome as opposed to burning pain symptomology of a known organic origin.

Figure 7.1 Chapter plan

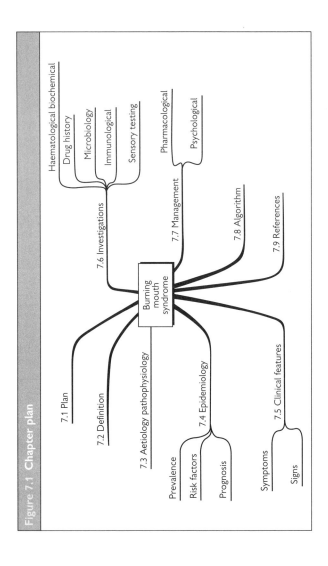

7.3 **Aetiology patho-physiology**

Any hypotheses about the pathophysiology of BMS should take into account three key features:

- Over-representation of menopausal women
- High prevalence of anxiety/depressive disorders among BMS patients
- Strictly oral location of the symptoms.

A first hypothesis proposes that each of these three key features of BMS may have their corresponding steroid changes. Menopause is associated with changes in gonadal steroids levels. The presence of chronic anxiety or post-traumatic chronic stress may provoke a functional impairment of the hypothalamic-pituitary-adrenal axis and lead to a dysregulation of the adrenal production of steroids. The restriction of the symptoms to the mouth is related to the synthesis of neuro-active steroids which can be site specific and confined in a very restricted area of the body.

The decrease in gonadal and neuroactive steroids and the loss of their neuroprotective effect, in combination with dysregulated adrenal steroid levels may result in the oral nerve terminal neurodegenerative changes that have been reported in histological studies of stomatodynia subjects.

A second hypothesis is focused on the frequent co-presentation of burning pain and dysgueusia. It proposes that neuropathic changes inside the taste nervous system induce the burning sensation by removing the inhibitory control on the somatic small fibre afferents responsible for the burning sensations. Anesthesia of the chorda tympani can intensify pain induced by capsaicin on the contralateral anterior tongue suggesting the presence of central inhibitory interactions between taste and oral pain. Furthermore, the intensification of pain was found to be related to an individual's genetic ability to taste PROP (6-n-propyl-thiouracil), with the greatest intensification found in 'supertasters' who report the bitterest sensation from PROP testing. Based on these taste/pain interactions, it is believed that BMS could also be the clinical manifestation of taste damage, to the chorda tympani, with consequent release of inhibition in the glossopharyngeal nerve (taste phantoms, alterations in touch and pain) and the trigeminal nerve (touch and pain changes). Consistent with this model, severe taste damage has been found on psychophysical testing in many BMS patients.

It is possible that the two hypotheses interact. Both clinical and physiological studies have demonstrated the effect of oestrogen on taste sensation, especially with respect to postmenopausal patients.

7.4 **Epidemiology**

7.4.1 **Prevalence/incidence**

An important factor in epidemiological studies presented in the literature is the choice of the sample, which may not be representative of the general population, and the varying methodology. This is emphasised in a study in which three different populations were sampled for comparison. For instance it was found that the prevalence of burning amongst patients attending a menopause, diabetic or general dental clinic was 26%, 10% and 2.6% respectively. The most common estimate is 1% of the general population.

7.4.2 **Risk factors**

Women are more frequently affected than are men, and the relative proportion is between three to twenty females for each male, depending on the study. Women affected are menopausal or post-menopausal and have an average age of approximately 60 years.

7.4.3 **Prognosis**

There are few studies documenting the long-term prognosis of BMS. Anecdotally, it has been observed that BMS is generally present over a number of years but there may be periods of remission. Spontaneous remission rates of 20% after 7 years or 3% after 5 years have been given.

7.5 **Clinical features**

The symptoms and signs are summarized in Figure 7.2

7.5.1 **Symptoms**

The most frequently affected areas are the tongue, palate and gingiva, lips and the pharynx. The pain is generally bilateral and symmetrical and usually appears independent of a nervous pathway. Pain intensity is variable between patients, ranging between simple irritation to the worst pain imaginable. The usual term patients use to describe the pain is simply 'burning' but they also describe abnormal sensations, and unlike some other neuropathic pain syndromes, there is usually no major paroxysmal component.

The burning pain usually occurs daily, is continuous throughout the day and tends to worsen over the day. Sleep disturbances may be reported as a parallel phenomenon but a causal relationship is unlikely, as loss of sleep is rarely due to the presence of pain. In some patients the burning pain may be triggered or exacerbated by certain foods, particularly if spicy or acidic. However, in most patients, food or drink alleviates the pain temporarily. The burning sensation is often accompanied by oral dysesthesia, and with a feeling of changes in saliva but usually without concurrent findings of objective xerostomia. Dysguesia is often reported, with patients experiencing taste phantoms such as bitter,

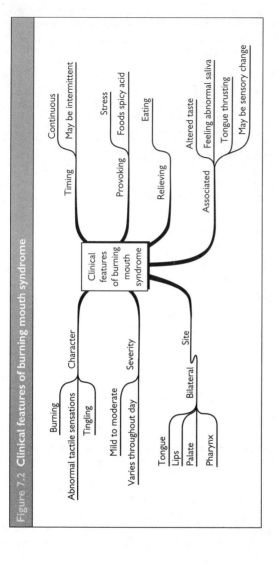

Figure 7.2 Clinical features of burning mouth syndrome

- Clinical features of burning mouth syndrome
  - Character
    - Burning
    - Abnormal tactile sensations
    - Tingling
  - Severity
    - Mild to moderate
    - Varies throughout day
  - Site
    - Bilateral
      - Tongue
      - Lips
      - Palate
      - Pharynx
  - Timing
    - Continuous
    - May be intermittent
  - Provoking
    - Stress
    - Foods spicy acid
  - Relieving
    - Eating
  - Associated
    - Altered taste
    - Feeling abnormal saliva
    - Tongue thrusting
    - May be sensory change

metallic or foul taste sensations, or sometimes dulling of taste sensation. Patients often present with high scores in psychometric scales associated with both depression and anxiety although no causal relationship has been found.

7.5.2 **Signs**

Usually no painful lesions are detected. However, it is not uncommon for BMS to co-present with generally painless and benign lesions such as geographic tongue or fissured tongue. It is unlikely that the pain is the result of these lesions since successful treatment of the lesions do not resolve the burning pain.

7.6 **Investigations**

Before a diagnosis of BMS is entertained, burning pain from a local or systemic cause should be ruled out as shown in Figure 7.3. This is mainly done through a series of investigations.

7.6.1 **Haematological and biochemical**

- Haemoglobin Vitamin B, folate and iron
- Glucose random and full glucose tolerance testing if indicated
- Urea, electrolytes, creatinine.

7.6.2 **Drug history**

Some medications such as angiotensin converting enzyme (ACE) inhibitors have been reported to be associated with burning pain.

7.6.3 **Microbiological**

- Herpes
- Candidiasis.

7.6.4 **Immunological tests appropriate for**

- Sjogren's Syndrome
- Systemic Lupus
- Allergy testing dental materials and dentures, and products such as toothpastes, mouth rinses and food constituents such as cinnamon.

7.6.5 **Sensory testing**

These are described in Chapter 3 but as yet are not clinically practical.

7.7 **Management**

The oral mucosa should be assessed and treated for tissue changes and lesions before burning mouth is considered. The treatment for BMS is pharmacological, with psychological support as detailed in Chapter 5, section 5.5. Surgical modalities are unlikely to be useful and over treatment may be harmful. Table 7.1 summarizes interventions that have been reported.

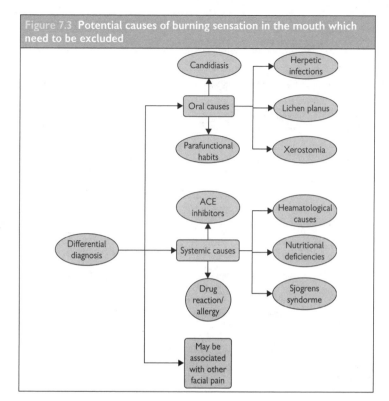

Figure 7.3 Potential causes of burning sensation in the mouth which need to be excluded

7.7.1 **Pharmacological therapies**

Only a few randomized, placebo-controlled trials (RCT) have been performed and only two clinically useful pharmacological treatments have shown to be significantly better than placebo, topical application of clonazepam and alpha-lipoic acid, an anti-oxidant nutritional supplement. Systemic capsaicin used in a short RCT has also been shown to be effective, but the numerous side effects make this treatment a less attractive option. These studies have not been replicated.

In an open label study, systemic clonazepam has also been reported to improve pain in approximately 70% of BMS patients. In the same study, there was reportedly a correlation between recent onset of pain and a positive response to therapy.

Other interventions have arisen from open-label studies and case reports, some echoing therapy used for other neuropathic pain syndromes and demonstrated varied outcomes. For example, tricyclic antidepressants (amytriptyline and clomipramine) have been tried for BMS, which reported a rather poor

Table 7.1 Management of burning mouth syndrome

Drug/therapy	Daily dose range	Efficacy NNT	Side effects	Comments
Proven in RCTs but in clinical practise limited effectiveness				
Antioxidant alphalipoic acid	600 mg then 200 mg after 20 days	NNT 1.6–3.3	Nil reported	Several studies from same centre, not all double blind
Cognitive behaviour therapy	One hour for 12–15 weeks	More effective than no treatment no NNT	Nil reported	Single blind
Clonazepam topical	1 mg sucked for 3 minutes	10/16 still some benefit at 6/12 no NNT	Nil significant	study 14 days, follow up 6 months
Benzydamine topical	0.15% solution 15 ml three times daily	Not effective	Nil	High quality RCT
Capsaicin systemic	0.25% capsule three times daily	NNT 1–2	Gastric pain in 32% increase over time	Poor randomisation, only used 30 days, side effects limit its use
Trazodone	200 mg daily	No effect	Drowsiness and dizziness	High quality RCT
Amisulpride Paroxetine Sertraline	50 mg daily 20 mg daily 50 mg daily	All effective no NNT	Mild non specific	No placebo
Commonly used but no RCT				
Clonazepam	0.25 mg–1 mg daily	Limited	Drowsiness	Use at night to avoid side effects
Gabapentin	300 mg–2400 mg daily	Limited	Ataxia, dizziness, drowsiness, nausea, headache, weight gain	
Pregablin	100–300 mg daily	May be effective	Dizziness, tiredness, headaches, weight gain	Used in neuropathic pain use twice daily

outcome with only 19% of the patients being improved. Despite strong side effects, antipsychotics such as amisulpride (50mg/day) or levosulpiride (100mg/day) have also been suggested. Anxiolytic drugs such as chlodiazepoxide (5–10 mg 3 times per day) or diazepam (6 to 15 mg per day) have also been advocated.

Studies concluded that there was no improvement after administration of gabapentin, mouthwash with benzydamine chlorhydrate, or trazodone, an antidepressant belonging to the specific serotonine reuptake inhibitor (SSRI) group. Finally, many topical treatments such as xylocaine gel, capsaicin cream, salivary substitute or systemic drugs such as tramadol and pregabalin are used, although there is little literature to support their use in BMS.

7.7.2 **Psychological interventions**

Reassurance that there is a physiological basis for the symptoms is very important and allows many patients to come to terms with their condition. Patients with BMS are often anxious about their symptoms, in part because of the absence of a proved organic cause and a known pathophysiology and there is some evidence that counseling may be helpful. One controlled study has shown that cognitive-behavioral therapy one hour per week for four mouths was successful in decreasing pain intensity.

Patient information in the form of a written leaflet as shown in the appendix is also helpful.

7.8 **Algorithm**

Management of BMS remains difficult as the interventions used in RCTS do not seem to be effective in clinical practise. The algorithm (Figure 7.4) therefore lists a wide range of interventions.

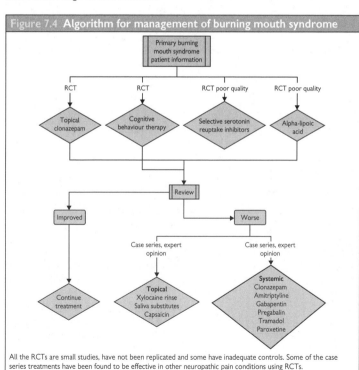

Figure 7.4 Algorithm for management of burning mouth syndrome

All the RCTs are small studies, have not been replicated and some have inadequate controls. Some of the case series treatments have been found to be effective in other neuropathic pain conditions using RCTs.

7.9 **References**

Bergdahl, J., Anneroth, G., Perris, H. (1995). Cognitive therapy in the treatment of patients with resistant burning mouth syndrome: a controlled study. *Journal of Oral Pathology and Medicine,* **24**: 213–15.

Buchanan, J.A., Zakrzewska, J.M. (2007). Burning mouth syndrome. *BMJ Clinical Evidence* 433–434. Website with full details http://www.clinicalevidence.bmj.com

Gremeau-Richard, C., Woda, A., Navez, M.L., Attal, N., Bouhassira, D., Gagnieu, M.C., Laluque, J.F., Picard, P., Pionchon, P., Tubert, S. (2004). Topical clonazepam in stomatodynia: A randomised placebo-controlled study. *Pain,* **108**: 51–7.

Grushka, M. (1987). Clinical features of burning mouth syndrome. *Oral Surgery Oral Medicine. Oral Pathology,* **63**: 30–6.

Patton, L.L., Siegel, M.A., Benoliel, R., De Laat, A. (2007). Management of burning mouth syndrome: systematic review and management recommendations. *Oral Surgery Oral Medicine Oral Pathology Oral Radiology Endodontics,* **103**: Suppl:S39.e1–13.

Scala, A., Checchi, L., Montevecchi, M., Marini, I., Giamberardino, M.A. (2003). Update on burning mouth syndrome: Overview and patient management. *Critical Review Oral Biology Medicine,* **14**: 275–91.

Zakrzewska, J.M., Forssell, H., Glenny, A.M. (2005). Interventions for the treatment of burning mouth syndrome. *Cochrane Database Systematic Reviews,* **25**(1): CD002779.

Chapter 8

Persistent idiopathic facial pain (atypical facial pain)

Thomas List and Charlotte Feinmann

Key points

- Persistent idiopathic facial pain comprises several different pain conditions. Atypical odontalgia may be a specific variant defined as 'a persistent chronic intraoral pain located in a region where a tooth had been endodontically or surgically treated (e.g. root canal filling, apicetomy, or extractions), in absence of any identifiable dental causes'
- Pain is only very loosely related to dental or TMJ pathology
- Important to avoid unnecessary investigations
- Sympathetic enquiry into how the pain interferes with the patient's life will reveal goals for improvement
- Early discussion and intervention may prevent the development of chronic symptoms
- Medications, reassurance, review.

8.1 Chapter plan

Figure 8.1 is an outline of the main contents of this chapter.

8.2 Definitions

The International Headache Society (2004) has defined 'persistent idiopathic facial pain' (PIFP) as:

(a) Pain in the face, presently daily and persistent for all or most of the the day, fulfilling criteria B and C.

(b) Pain is confined at onset to a limited area on one side of the face, and deep and poorly localized.

Figure 8.1 Chapter plan

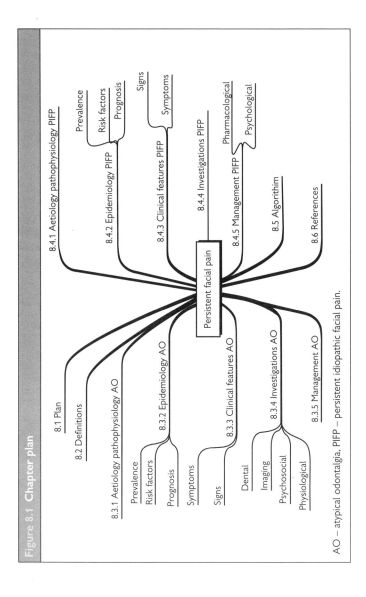

AO – atypical odontalgia, PIFP – persistent idiopathic facial pain.

(c) Pain is not associated with sensory loss or other physical signs.

(d) Investigations including X-ray of the face and jaws do not demonstrate any relevant abnormality.

Previously used terms for PIFP are atypical facial pain (AFP), atypical odontalgia (AO), phantom tooth pain, and idiopathic toothache. The International Headache Society definition of persistent idiopathic facial pain comprises several different pain conditions. AO is defined as 'a continuous pain in the teeth or in a tooth socket after extraction in the absence of any identifiable dental cause.' Often there is also a history of frequent restorative, endodontic procedures or it is a site of extractions and yet there are no physical or radiographic findings to explain the pain.

AFP is a poorly localized persistent pain in the face and it may be an idiopathic (somatoform) pain syndrome, where the face and the mouth may be included in the pain description. PIFP and AO, share some characteristics with temporomandibular disorders (TMD) but differ significantly in report of dental trauma, jaw function, pain duration, and pain localization. Further research is needed to explain the pain-related mechanisms and evidence-based criteria for PIFP and whether subgroups within the classification are necessary.

There is considerable overlap between PIFP and AO, the latter being much more localized, so these will be described separately with a greater emphasis on AO for which there is more research. It is also unclear as yet whether AO is the same as trigeminal neuropathic pain or trigeminal neuropathy and the former is described in Chapter 11 section 11.2.

8.3 Atypical odontalgia

8.3.1 Aetiology and pathophysiology of AO

Some researchers suggest that, without known aetiologic factors, AO is best viewed as an idiopathic pain condition but it may have both psychological and neuropathic origins.

Nerve injury that occurs in relation to invasive dental treatment, such as endodontic procedures or tooth extraction, was suggested to be associated with the development of persistent neuropathic orofacial pain as most AO patients relate the onset of pain to invasive dental treatment such as endodontic procedures or tooth extraction.

In summary, significant abnormalities in intra-oral somatosensory function that are often found may reflect peripheral and central sensitization of trigeminal pathways. At present, the main hypothesis in the literature is that AO is a neuropathic condition, but this is unconfirmed and hence its inclusion as. trigeminal neuropathic pain in Chapter 11 section 11.2.

8.3.2 Epidemiology

Information on the prevalence and incidence of AO is limited. In retrospective studies, AO was estimated to be present in 3%–6% of clinical cases undergoing endodontic treatment. Both sexes and all adult ages can be affected but most are women in their late 40s. The higher ratio of females to males is similar to the ratios reported for other orofacial pain conditions.

Postulated risk factors: chronic pain, pain intensity, and previous episodes of painful treatments.

Prognosis: There are no systematic, longitudinal epidemiological studies on PIFP or AO so whether it is life-long is unknown.

8.3.3 **Clinical features**

8.3.3.1 *Symptoms*

Most AO patients report persistent, moderately intense intra-oral pain that often had an onset in conjunction with dental treatment.

The intra-oral pain site in AO is often well localized and can include any tooth or mucosa of an extraction site, but the pain may move from tooth to tooth following dental procedures. Although the most common sites are the molars and premolars in the upper jaw, the incisors are also nearly as frequently involved.

Self-reported pain intensity and use of pain descriptors are similar in AO and TMD. The McGill Pain Questionnaire (MPQ) is therefore unable to distinguish between these conditions.

It has been found that these patients report psychological distress with mean depression and somatization being higher than the general population.

AO often results in repeated and possibly unnecessary dental measures such as root canal treatments, apicetomies, and extractions – a vicious cycle of treatment visits to numerous health-care professionals is common. In some case reports, all teeth have undergone root canal treatment and apicetomies. The key features are summarized in Figure 8.2.

8.3.3.2 *Signs*

Somatosensory changes in AO patients such as hyperesthesia at the pain site, allodynia, and exacerbation of pain evoked by temperature have been reported in several studies. About two-thirds of patients with AO develop TMD.

8.3.4 **Investigations**

8.3.4.1 *Dental*

The most useful diagnostic methods in patients with PIFP are history taking and somatosensory testing. Several pain conditions have been suggested to mimic AO and are important to rule out before making a diagnosis of AO. Pulpal pain conditions are probably the most difficult differential diagnoses to rule out, for others please see Chapter 6.

The diagnostic work-up is provided in Chapter 2. Examination of the masticatory system and cervical spine may provide information for excluding TMD and referred pain from the cervical region.

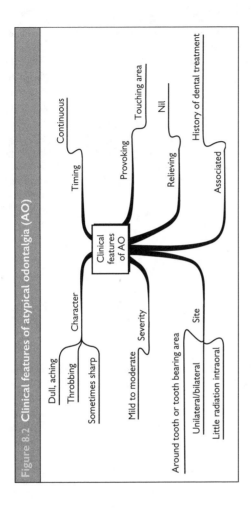

Figure 8.2 Clinical features of atypical odontalgia (AO)

Clinical features of AO

- Timing
  - Continuous
- Provoking
  - Touching area
- Relieving
  - Nil
- Associated
  - History of dental treatment
- Character
  - Dull, aching
  - Throbbing
  - Sometimes sharp
- Severity
  - Mild to moderate
- Site
  - Around tooth or tooth bearing area
  - Unilateral/bilateral
  - Little radiation intraoral

Simple diagnostic procedures such as the use of local anaesthetic (LA) blocks help in understanding the clinical manifestation of a painful condition. Patients with AO complaints may demonstrate a wide range of responses to topical anaesthesia or LA blocks, for example, complete, partial, or no pain reduction to somatosensory blocks.

8.3.4.2 *Imaging*

Radiographic examinations of the jaws and teeth should include conventional radiographs: panoramic and periapical radiographs. Preliminary findings indicate that cone beam computed tomography (CBCT) and magnetic resonance imaging (MRI) may provide more information than conventional radiography in the examination and diagnosis of intra-oral orofacial pain conditions – see Chapter 3.

8.3.4.3 *Physiological*

Somatosensory assessment includes bedside neurological qualitative and quantitative sensory testing – see Chapter 3.

8.3.4.4 *Psychological*

Several studies support an association between AO and different psychological conditions such as depression, somatoform pain disorder, and anxiety so these should be assessed as described in Chapter 3.

Cases of excessive dental treatment are rare, and it may be that pain behaviour in these individuals differs from the vast majority of AO patients, and is related more to personality traits rather than to pain.

8.3.5 **Management**

Few randomized, controlled trials that evaluate the treatment effect in AO have been conducted. There is one systematic review which emphasises the lack of evidence for effective treatment options. Overall, this group of patients is difficult to treat. They often need much help, support, and resources. Pharmacologic treatment has seldom had a very good effect, and often only a small to moderate reduction of pain is achievable. Management is the same as for PIFP and this is discussed in the next section.

There is no evidence that surgical procedures would improve the pain condition. Most probably, repeated operations will increase hyperexcitability in the area.

8.4 **Persistent idiopathic facial pain**

8.4.1 **Aetiology and pathophysiology of PIFP**

This is best viewed as an idiopathic pain condition. There is also the association between chronic facial pain and several psychological factors but the aetiology remains largely unknown.

8.4.2 **Epidemiology**

Facial pain affects between 10–15% of the general population but not all patients seek help.

Those that seek help consult on average 7 professionals, including dentists; general medical practitioners; neurologists; ear, nose, and throat (ENT) specialists; maxillofacial surgeons; psychiatrists; ophthalmologists; and dermatologists.

Risk: PIFP is rather poorly understood and it is unclear why some individuals are more vulnerable to trauma or iatrogenic damage than other. Risk factors may be:

- History of widespread pain
- Genetic susceptibility
- Female sex
- Passive coping traits.

Prognosis: There is little understanding of prognosis in these patients but growing evidence for psychological distress as a consequence rather than a cause of pain, and this distress is likely to contribute to the persistence of symptoms.

Poor quality of life will increase persistence of symptoms as the following often occur:

- Decreased social activities because of fatigue
- Reduced capacity to eat in public due to difficulty in mouth opening and altered taste
- Altered mood, speech, self-image, and digestion.

Treatment is most likely to be effective when the pain history is short. Successful treatment of facial pain of many years' duration is a much greater challenge. However, improvement is only sustained when an attempt is made to resolve psychological problems. It is not clear who responds to what treatment, or indeed what problems actually need to be treated.

8.4.3 **Clinical features**

The key clinical features are shown in Figure 8.3. The pain is usually poorly localized and perceived as arising from the muscles of the face and jaw, although increased EMG activity does not correlate with pain.

Patients also report pain that radiates all over the head and neck and down to the arms, as well as general aches and pain. Symptoms wax and wane in intensity over days and weeks. Cold weather, psychological stresses and dental treatment may all make things worse.

It is not unusual for patients with chronic facial pain to have a number of other problems:

- Irritable bowel syndrome
- Headache
- Neck ache
- Back ache

Figure 8.3 Clinical features of persistent idiopathic facial pain (PIFP)

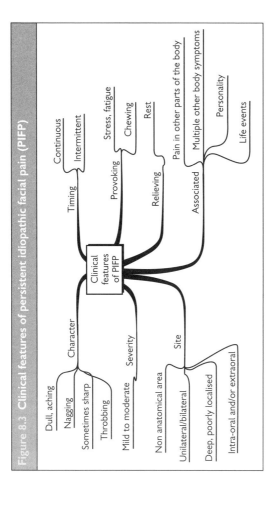

- Dysmenorrhoea
- Pruritis
- Cold intolerance
- Cognitive dysfunction
- Multiple sensitivities
- Dizziness.

About 50% of patients with chronic facial pain also complain of chronic fatigue and about 50%–70% of pain patients suffer from sleep disturbance. In general those with long-standing pain can continue normal activities, despite the pain being a daily or near daily occurrence. Recent evidence suggests that it may be more helpful to assess patients in terms of what the patients are told and what they understand about their problems.

8.4.4 **Investigations**

It is crucial to understand that patients are extensively investigated and frequently off-loaded from specialist to specialist in search of a diagnosis. Patients feel ill-understood and over-investigated. Assessment of disability may lead to more precise treatment guidelines. Sympathetic inquiry by the practitioner will help to assess the level of interference with the patient's life and provide a record against which subsequent improvement may be gauged. These are described in Chapter 3.

8.4.5 **Management**

It has been suggested that emphasis should be put on therapist-patient communication and that effective communication during the early phases of facial pain can prevent the development of long-term problems. Doctors and dentists should be aware of the importance of listening to the patient's beliefs about their pain, and of trying to address their concerns without resorting to outdated psychogenic models of pain. Reassurance about the non-malignant nature of chronic pain is also important, but empty promises that 'things will get better' are unhelpful. The message is that talking to patients is often more useful, albeit sometimes more demanding, than operating on them. It is important to try and prevent acute pain becoming chronic and prevention of excessive dentistry in part prevents central sensitization.

8.4.6 **Pharmacological**

The major drugs used are summarized in Table 8.1 below. Anticonvulsant drugs have long been used in pain management of central and peripheral neuropathic pain conditions but no study has included patients with PIFP.

In systematic reviews, evidence for the pain-relieving effect of topical capsaicin cream and lidocaine patches was found in the treatment of neuropathic pain conditions but little information is available for AO and PIFP. Since topical administration has the advantage of no systematic effect, these drugs may be used during a test period to evaluate whether the pain relief they provide is sufficient.

Table 8.1 Management of persistent idiopathic facial pain/atypical odontalgia

Drug/therapy	Daily dose range	Efficacy	Side effects
Amitriptyline	10–150 mg	Good	Nil reported but causes drowsiness, dry mouth
Dothiepin included biteguard	25–150 mg	Likely to be effective insufficient evidence for biteguard	Drowsiness, dry mouth, dizziness
Fluoxetine	20 mg	Good	Nil reported but causes postural hypotension, sleep disturbance
Phenelzine	45 mg	Improved both pain and associated depression	Nil reported but causes postural hypotension, dizziness, insomnia, dry mouth
Sumatriptan	6 mg sc	Limited	
Venlafaxine	75 mg	Limited	Commonest fatigue, loss of appetite, nausea, dry mouth
CBT with or without tricyclic antidepressants	6–12 sessions	High	If use drugs drowsiness, dryness
Information and reassurance		High	

8.4.7 **Psychological/non-medical**

Information to the patient about possible causes of the pain is an important part of treatment. An explanation of central and peripheral sensitisation may help patients understand why they are experiencing pain and abnormal sensory phenomena despite lack of radiographic pathology. Further details are provided in Chapter 5 Section 5.5.

The use of cognitive behavioural therapy in the management of chronic orofacial pain has been recommended. The purpose of cognitive behavioural therapy is to improve patients' knowledge and awareness of factors that influence the pain, and to help patients cope with their situation, learning to live with pain.

Some patients with severe idiopathic orofacial pain should be referred to a multidisciplinary pain team as they require complex clinical psychological or psychiatric treatment.

The majority of patients will respond to simple and inexpensive interventions especially if conservative intervention is offered in the early stages as chronic problems become much more difficult and costly to remedy.

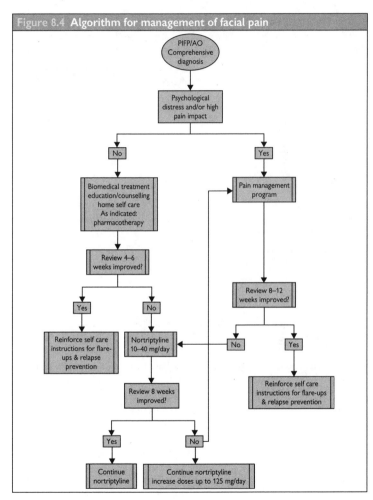

8.5 **Algorithm**

This is shown in figure 8.4. Although nortriptyline has not been evaluated in an RCT in chronic facial pain it is used in preference to amitriptyline as it causes less oral dryness.

Figure 8.4 Algorithm for management of facial pain

PIFP/AO
Comprehensive
diagnosis

Psychological
distress and/or high
pain impact

No

Yes

Biomedical treatment
education/counselling
home self care
As indicated:
pharmacotherapy

Pain management
program

Review 4–6
weeks improved?

Yes

No

Review 8–12
weeks improved?

Reinforce self care
instructions for flare-
ups & relapse
prevention

Nortriptyline
10–40 mg/day

No

Yes

Review 8 weeks
improved?

Reinforce self care
instructions for flare-ups
& relapse prevention

Yes

No

Continue
nortriptyline

Continue nortriptyline
increase doses up to 125 mg/day

8.6 **References**

Baad-Hansen, L. (2008). Atypical odontalgia – pathophysiology and clinical management. *Journal Oral Rehabilitation*, **35**: 1–11.

Feinmann, C. (1983). Psychogenic facial pain: presentation and treatment. *Journal Psychosomatic Research*, **27**: 403–10.

Feinmann, C., Newton-John, T. (2004). Psychiatric and psychological management considerations associated with nerve damage and neuropathic trigeminal pain. *Journal of Orofacial Pain*, **18**: 360–5.

Forssell, H., Tasmuth, T., Tenovuo, O., Hampf, G., Kalso, E. (2004). Venlafaxine in the treatment of atypical facial pain: a randomized controlled trial. *Journal of Orofacial Pain*, **18**: 131–7.

Lang, E., Kaltenhauser, M., Seidler, S., Mattenklodt, P., Neundorfer, B. (2005). Persistent idiopathic facial pain exists independent of somatosensory input from the painful region: findings from quantitative sensory functions and somatotopy of the primary somatosensory cortex. *Pain*, **118**: 80–91.

List, T., Axelsson, S., Leijon, G. (2003). Pharmacologic interventions in the treatment of temporomandibular disorders, atypical facial pain, and burning mouth syndrome. A qualitative systematic review. *Journal of Orofacial Pain*, **17**: 301–10.

List, T., Leijon, G., Helkimo, M., Öster, A., Dworkin, S.F., Svensson, P. (2007). Clinical Findings and Psychosocial Factors in Patients with Atypical Odontalgia: A Case-Control Study. *Journal of Orofacial Pain*, **21**: 89–98.

List, T., Leijon, G., Helkimo, M., Öster, A., Svensson, P. (2006). Effect of local anesthesia on atypical odontalgia – a randomized controlled trial. *Pain*, **122**: 306–14.

Pigg, M., Petersson, A., Petersson, K., Maly, P., List, T. (2006). A comparative analysis of MRI, CBCT and conventional radiography in patients with atypical odontalgia and symptomatic apical peridontitis: preliminary results. *Swedish Dental Journal,* **4**: abstr. 4.

Polycarpou, N., Ng, Y.L., Canavan, D., Moles, D.R., Gulabivala, K. (2005). Prevalence of persistent pain after endodontic treatment and factors affecting its occurrence in cases with complete radiographic healing. *International Endodontics Journal*, **38**: 169–78.

Woda, A., Tubert-Jeannin, S., Bouhassira, D., Attal, N., Fleiter, B., Goulet, J.P., Gremeau-Richard, C., Navez, M.L., Picard, P., Pionchon, P., Albuisson, E. (2005). Towards a new taxonomy of idiopathic orofacial pain. *Pain*, **116**: 396–406.

Chapter 9

Temporomandibular disorders (TMD)

Heli Forssell and Richard Ohrbach

> **Key points**
>
> - TMD is a musculoskeletal disorder with primary symptoms of pain localized to the face and temple and limitation in mandibular function
> - Physical, psychological, and genetic factors have a bearing on the onset and maintenance of TMD
> - Diagnostics should include both physical and psychosocial factors. The clinical examination confirms regional pain from movement or palpation, limitation of mobility, and/or interference in function. A screening model is used for the psychosocial domain
> - Treatment is tailored to pain and patient characteristics, and management using symptomatic treatments with an emphasis on self care is dominant
> - Different treatment modalities result in comparable treatment outcomes and most patients respond favorably to simple noninvasive treatments
> - When treating patients with high-pain impact and/or psychosocial distress, a more comprehensive management strategy is mandatory.

9.1 Chapter plan

Figure 9.1 is an outline of the main contents of this chapter.

9.2 Definition

TMD (temporomandibular disorders), a collective term referring to a classification of musculoskeletal disorders affecting the masticatory muscles and/or the temporomandibular joints (TMJs), is usually subdivided into three major categories:
- myofascial pain disorder

Figure 9.1 Chapter plan

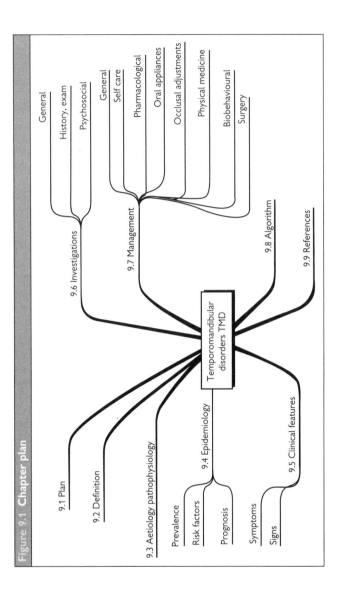

- TMJ disc interference disorders which are further separated into
  - disc displacement with reduction, characterized by jaw-movement related clicks or pops which are associated with asynchronous movement of the disk relative to the condylar head
  - disc displacement without reduction, characterized by permanent displacement of the disk. In acute form this causes limited jaw opening and TMJ pain, but over time pain free function is usually regained.
- TMJ degenerative joint disease, termed osteoarthrosis when pain free, and termed osteoarthritis when associated with clinical pain of variable intensity and restricted jaw movements.

Although myofascial pain is the most prevalent form of TMDs, multiple diagnoses involving both muscle and joints are common.

9.3 **Aetiology and pathophysiology**

Aside from direct trauma, aetiology for TMD appears to involve multiple intersecting factors which vary from person to person. Factors that appear to modify host resistance include:

- Widespread pain
- Genetic vulnerability for pain sensitivity
- Female hormones
- Passive coping traits
- Embedded illness models.

More proximal factors such as sleep bruxism, other parafunctional behaviours, and unilateral chewing appear to be capable of triggering a TMD episode. The pathophysiology of the individual diagnostic TMDs is summarized as follows.

9.3.1 **Myofascial pain disorder**

This is a regional masticatory muscle disorder, believed to be functional in nature, aggravated by overuse of the muscles and perpetuated by such overuse. When overt trauma is the cause, the disorder is self-limiting but many factors in addition to overuse contribute to chronicity. Consequently, early treatment that sufficiently addresses the pain itself is important. When myofascial pain becomes chronic, psychophysiologic activation of motor units appears to be a significant factor for maintaining the disorder.

9.3.2 **Disk disorders**

There are 4 identified stages:
1. simple displacement with reduction and without functional impairment
2. simple displacement with intermittent locking and interference
3. displacement without reduction and with substantial functional impairment in function
4. displacement without reduction and with relatively complete functional recovery.

While there is obviously a progression in that later stages evolves from earlier stages, little is known about factors that promote progression. In contrast, the vast majority of simple displacements do not progress, and the long-term outcomes indicate relatively good recovery for those that do progress which underlies the adequacy of symptomatic treatments.

9.3.3 **Degenerative joint changes**

The mechanisms underlying degenerative joint changes are believed to be the same for the TMJ as for other joints, and while some believe that disk displacements represent a risk factor for degenerative changes, there is equivalent data supporting the reverse causation. One unique factor regarding the TMJ is that it appears to exhibit adaptive changes throughout the lifespan in response to changes in the local environment (e.g. sleep-bruxism, loss of teeth) and so changes in joint morphology, per se, are not necessarily of concern.

9.3.4 **Progression from acute to chronic**

This is largely influenced by psychosocial factors and not by pathophysiological ones other than the pathophysiology underlying pain itself. Available evidence suggests that it is the individual's response to the pain that drives the expression of the behavioural factors. Simultaneously, central nervous system (CNS) plasticity leads to alterations in the pain system itself shifting the genesis of the pain from purely peripheral mechanisms to also include central mechanisms. Behavioural changes to the pain further amplify these CNS changes to include alteration in other systems (e.g. mood, anxiety, treatment-seeking). Consequently, it is the pathophysiology of TMD as a whole that is more challenging and perhaps useful in terms of management.

Specifically, muscle and/or TMJ pain and/or joint interferences can produce significant impact on the individual in terms of adaptive behaviours (e.g. to avoid the pain, to make a dysfunctional joint work better). While such behaviours can be truly 'adaptive' in the short term, their continual presence leads to further compensatory adaptations resulting in extension of a TMD into the cervical region with subsequent expression of pain and limitation there as well, and the continued 'adaptive' behaviours appear to increase the likelihood of persistent pain.

In summary, addressing pain and restoring normal function during the acute stage is the presently understood hallmark for treatment, and it remains the cornerstone of management for the chronic stage as well.

9.4 **Epidemiology**

9.4.1 **Prevalence/incidence**

TMDs are the most common cause of non dental pain in the orofacial region:
- prevalence figures range from 4% to 12% in adult population
- the incidence of new onset TMD pain varies from 1.6% to 3.9% per year
- TMD pain is about twice as common in adult women as in men

- TMD pain becomes more prevalent in the teenage years, peaks in the middle years, and declines into old age.

9.4.2 **Risk factors**

These are shown in Figure 9.2.

In addition, certain occlusal characteristics may have weak associations and may contribute to the burden imposed by other risk factors.

9.4.3 **Prognosis**

- Signs and symptoms of TMD often fluctuate, may be transient and self-limiting, and can typically be resolved without serious long-term morbidity. This also applies to cases with structural hard or soft tissue changes, i.e. osteoarthritis/arthrosis and disc displacements
- While most TMD pains can be easily managed, a minority of patients, usually less than 20%, may have persistent pain. Depression, somatisation, and other psychological factors as well as pain in other body sites have been shown to predict continuation or worsening of TMD pain.

9.5 **Clinical features**

The clinical features are summarized in Figure 9.3.

9.5.1 **Symptoms**

The primary symptom is regional pain, which is modified by jaw functions such as rest vs. chewing. Because pain fluctuates, a prior time frame such as one month is generally used in order to provide current diagnosis. Reports of joint clicking-type sounds are common, but clicks alone are seldom a cause for concern.

In contrast indicators of degenerative changes would be a combination of

- Clicking
- Limitation of movement – full-open locking, partial open locking,
- Momentary hesitation in opening
- Sudden inability to fully close the teeth
- Crepitus.

Associated symptoms take two forms: the first includes other somatic symptoms such as ear pain, fullness of the ear, or alterations in normal sensation such as dysesthesias, and the second includes psychosocial symptoms such as pain exacerbations being linked to psychosocial stress.

9.5.2 **Signs**

Deviations and/or restriction in movement and pain sensitivity to palpation are the most common. Detectable TMJ noises, via palpation or auscultation, are common but unreliable due to poor stability of the noises.

Figure 9.2 Risk factors for temporomandibular disorders (TMD) showing those supported by good quality evidence and those for which there is as yet insufficient evidence

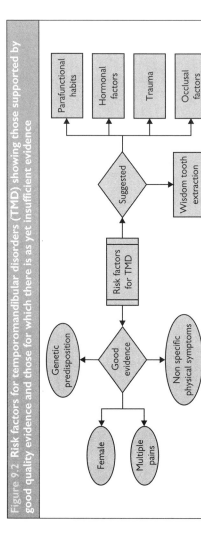

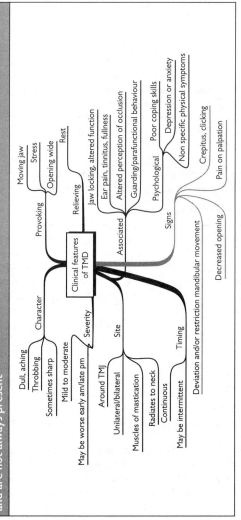

Figure 9.3 Clinical features of temporomandibular disorders (TMD). Not all these features need to be present to make the diagnosis. The psychosocial factors are shown under the associated features and are not always present

9.6 Investigations

9.6.1 General

Pain disorder diagnoses emerge from the history, and the clinical examination confirms signs consistent with the pain disorder. The examination is also used to rule out other competing diagnoses such as odontogenic problems. The description here pertains to the procedures for assessing TMD, and material should be sought elsewhere for necessary tests for other disorders. Because the clinical findings fluctuate and are relatively soft as objective findings, standardized clinical examination procedures are preferred such as structured examination directions and standardized palpation forces. These procedures are described in the RDC/TMD which is a dual axis system including the physical findings and diagnosis and the psychosocial assessment. Further information regarding the RDC/TMD protocol can be found at http://www.rdc-tmdinternational.org.

9.6.2 History and clinical examination

The primary characteristic of a musculoskeletal pain disorder is the report of regional pain affected by rest, movement, or both. Diagnostic questions emerge when the pain extends beyond the masticatory system, when it does not follow anatomic patterns, and when temporal and quality characteristics are more related to other sources such as teeth. The temporal characteristics of TMD pain with respect to patterns within a day are believed to be important with respect to whether sleep bruxism, whether waking parafunction, both or neither are important causes. Pain patterning over a longer course (e.g. a week) is often more complicated, increasing the complexity of using temporal characteristics as firm diagnostic guidelines. Co-morbidity with other pain disorders (typically, headaches or cervical pain) is assessed in terms of initial onset of the respective disorders, onset of episodes of each pain, and progression over time. The history should also assess mechanical problems with jaw function in order to discover whether jaw locking of any type is present or was present in the past (i.e. displacement without reduction, now with normal mobility).

The clinical examination includes general inspection: symmetry of development, presence of scars (i.e. prior trauma), and alterations in motor function. The opening pattern and extent of pain-free and maximal opening are assessed, and any pain produced with opening is noted. Pain sensitivity to palpation of the masticatory muscles and TMJs is performed, and while graded responses can be obtained simple reports of yes/no seem sufficient for diagnostic purposes. Palpation forces of about 1 kg seem sufficient for the masseter and temporalis muscles and 0.5 kg for the remaining muscles and TMJs. Joint sounds can be assessed with either auscultation or palpation; the former is more sensitive but also increases false positive risk. Orthopaedic tests of muscle and joint function can be performed but the diagnostic yield beyond that of palpation appears to be minimal.

9.6.3 **Additional tests**
- Panoramic radiography is considered standard as a first stage evaluation; it provides important information for differential diagnosis of tooth pathology and other bony pathology, and provides a gross assessment of the TMJs
- CT may be warranted if panoramic radiography positive
- MRI for disc pathology – its use should be balanced with recognition that displacements with reduction, in the absence of locking or interference, seldom require treatment
- Other tests advocated for diagnosis, such as EMG and jaw movement studies, have insufficient supporting evidence to warrant their use.

9.6.4 **Psychosocial assessment**
All patients with TMD, whether acute or chronic, should be assessed at this level.

Depression, anxiety, non-specific physical symptoms (sometimes referred to as somatisation), functional limitation of the jaw, and pain-related disability are often present and can be assessed via a range of instruments used in medical settings as discussed in Chapter 3, and are conveniently included in the RDC/TMD which can be found at http://www.rdc-tmdinternational.org in a variety of languages.

These constructs should be assessed in two ways:
- Standardized self-report instruments prior to the clinical interview
- During the interview based on the information obtained from the self-report instrument.

This permits an efficient and more reliable assessment of these constructs. Positive findings indicate caution regarding the possible need for further assessment and/or immediate inclusion of behavioural interventions into treatment, depending on other aspects of the history.

9.7 **Management**

The following evidence is available:
- Systematic reviews in the Cochrane Library
- Several systematic or evidence-based reviews in peer reviewed journals.

9.7.1 **General**
Because of the limited understanding of the pathogenesis and aetiology of TMD, management, rather than cure, is central just as for most other musculoskeletal conditions. The general goal of management is to alleviate pain and restore normal jaw functions. Immediate pain relief is an important treatment goal in order to avoid peripheral or central sensitization.

Treatments should be tailored to pain and patient characteristics as these can be important for potential poor treatment response and/or relapse.

The following needs to be taken into account:

• Physical symptoms
• Psychosocial status of the patients
• Pain-related limitations
• The impact of pain
• Chronicity
• Presence of widespread pain or other pain conditions
• Co-morbid disorders (e.g. sleep disturbances, non-specific somatic symptoms in other body systems).

Treatment response should in all cases be reviewed at 4–6 week intervals.

Various biomedical treatment modalities result in comparable treatment outcomes. This highlights the use of non-invasive, reversible management strategies instead of invasive, irreversible approaches. The fact that different treatments give similar results also allows patient preferences to be taken into consideration when selecting treatment approaches. Providing patients with comprehensive information about their symptoms and self-management strategies is essential in order for the patient to take an active role in the rehabilitation process.

In acute and subacute cases patient education, tailored exercise programmes, pain medication, and possible intraoral splint therapy are usually sufficient interventions. However, comprehensive management incorporating cognitive-behavioural methods, which emphasize self-management and the acquisition of self-control over the pain symptoms, have been shown to provide long-lasting benefits that exceed those observed with the usual clinical treatment for TMD. Comprehensive management is always essential when treating patients with pain-related impairments (dysfunctional patients). In chronic TMDs, a team approach in management, usually consisting of a dentist, psychologist, and a physiotherapist, is recommended. The main treatments are summarised in Table 9.1 and the algorithm in Figure 9.4.

9.7.2 **Self-care**

An empowered patient usually does better than being a passive recipient of treatment. TMD self-care programmes usually incorporate

• Use of cold and hot packs
• Automassage
• Various jaw exercises
• Over the counter pain medications
• Education about parafunctional jaw activities
• General relaxation skills.

Recent large RCTs showed self-care to be as effective in reducing symptoms and signs of TMD as intraoral splint therapy, and that structured self-care intervention produced longer lasting benefits compared to usual dental TMD treatments.

9.7.3 **Pharmacologic approaches**

See Table 9.1. With the exception of tricyclic antidepressants and possibly gabapentin for chronic TMD, pharmacological therapy is recommended for only short-term use in acute TMJ (NSAIDs) or muscle pain (muscle relaxants, benzodiazepines). Sufficient treatment of nociception can help prevent pain from becoming chronic.

In addition to systemic medications, intra-articular glucocorticosteroid injections have been used in patients with acute synovitis, but the evidence for efficacy comes mainly from injections of joints other than the TMJs.

9.7.4 **Appliances**

Different types of oral appliances have been used to treat both muscular and arthrogenous TMD symptoms. The most common and most rigorously studied is the full coverage stabilization appliance. The use of other types of appliances, such as partial coverage appliances and mandibular repositioning appliances, has declined, in part due to the lack of evidence supporting their efficacy and in part due to potential complications such as permanent changes in the occlusion.

In contrast to one RCT comparing the efficacy of stabilization splint to that of a non-occluding 'placebo' splint, several recent RCTs have provided evidence for modest therapeutic effects by splint therapy. Patients with regional myofascial pain respond more favourably to splint therapy compared to those with widespread pain. Stabilization splints have been shown to be as effective as acupuncture and some other physical medicine methods and biofeedback in decreasing TMD symptoms. Soft stabilization splints work equally well as hard acrylic splints, at least in the short term.

Table 9.1 Management of TMD

Category	Therapy	Efficacy/Evidence
Self care	Mixture of cold/hot packs, jaw exercises, reduction of parafunctional jaw activities	Effective/Large RCT
Pharmacological	NSAIDs Benzodiazepines Cyclobenzaprine Tricyclic antidepressants Gabapentin	Effective/2 RCTs Equivocal evidence Possibly effective/1 RCT Possibly effective/2 small RCTs Possibly effective/1 RCT
Oral appliances	Hard or soft stabilisation splints	Effective/several positive RCTs, one negative
Occlusal treatments	Occlusal adjustment	No evidence for efficacy
Physical medicine	Acupuncture Low level laser, TENS, ultrasound, thermal remedies, jaw manipulation	Equivocal evidence No evidence for efficacy
Biobehavioural	Cognitive behavioural therapy	Effective, several RCTs
Surgery	Arthrocentesis, arthroscopic surgery, open joint surgery	No evidence

The mode of action of the splint therapy is not well understood and there could be a variety of mechanisms:

• As behaviour-changing device
• Decreasing muscle activity and bruxism
• Changing maxillomandibular relationships.

Splints are also used to protect teeth from abrasive wear. Stabilization splints are worn during sleep. Splints should be adjusted as needed in order to maintain equal contacts on all of the teeth so that during any clenching, the forces are distributed equally to each tooth and the joints. The appliances are used until the symptoms subside. In cases of heavy bruxism splints can be in long term use and require periodic replacement.

9.7.5 Occlusal adjustment

Occlusal treatments for TMD have a long history in dentistry, but the current understanding of the mechanisms of TMD pain questions the association between occlusion and TMD. In particular, based on epidemiologic data and systematic studies, the relationship between occlusal interferences and TMD is considered weak, and there is insufficient evidence for the efficacy of occlusal adjustment in the treatment of TMD symptoms. For these reasons and because perceived changes in occlusion can be a consequence of TMD rather than the cause of the problem, occlusal therapy is in general not considered an appropriate treatment option for TMD.

9.7.6 Physical medicine

Acupuncture, low-level laser therapy, transcutaneous electrical nerve stimulation (TENS), ultrasound, thermal therapies, jaw manipulation and exercise are used to treat TMD symptoms, but high quality evidence is not available. Medium quality RCTs report similar outcomes for acupuncture vs. appliance therapy.

9.7.7 Biobehavioural interventions

These are discussed in Chapter 5, section 5.5 and may be the most crucial for long term management. The primary biobehavioural intervention is structured self-care, which shifts responsibility to the patient, provides important data for monitoring the potential importance of any related biobehavioural factors, and improves relapse resistance. If biobehavioural factors are critical, referral for pain-psychology evaluations is appropriate.

Further biobehavioural treatment consists of structured cognitive-behavioural treatment for pain, which includes

• Addressing treatment adherence
• General relaxation skills and their application to stress reactivity
• Pain cognitions and self-defeating behaviours
• Effective communication of body symptoms within good doctor-patient relationships
• Plans for managing flare-ups in the future.

Significant depression warrants additional evaluation for possible adjunctive medications.

9.7.8 Indications for TMJ surgery

Surgical interventions should be considered in cases with accurate diagnosis involving specific changes and symptoms in TMJ which have been refractory to appropriate nonsurgical therapies. The increased understanding of the molecular mechanisms of TMJ disc interference disorders and osteoarthritis may indicate a role for arthrocentesis in the early stages of TMD management. However, better designed trials are needed to determine the true benefit of all types of surgical treatments for TMD.

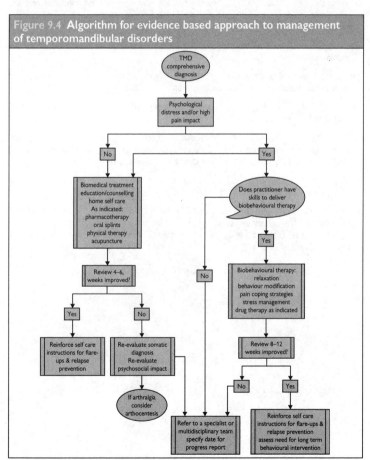

Figure 9.4 Algorithm for evidence based approach to management of temporomandibular disorders

9.8 Algorithm

The algorithm in Figure 9.4 provides a possible evidence based approach to the initial management of TMD and instructions for more complicated cases.

9.9 Key References

Diatchenko, L., Nackley, A.G., Slade, G.D., Fillingim, R.B., Maixner, W. (2006). Idiopathic pain disorders – pathways of vulnerability. *Pain*, **123**: 226–30.

Dworkin, S., LeResche, L., (1992). Research diagnostic criteria for temporomandibular disorders: review, criteria, examinations and specifications, critique. *Journal Craniomandibular Disorders and Facial Oral Pain*, **77**: 301–55.

Greene, C.S. (2001). The etiology of temporomandibular disorders: Implications for treatment. *Journal Orofacial Pain*, **25**: 93–105.

Laskin, M., Greene, C.S., Hylander, W.L. (eds) (2006). *TMDs. An evidence based approach to diagnosis and treatment*. Quintessence Publishing Co, Singapore.

Ren, K., Dubner, R. (1999). Central nervous system plasticity and persistent pain. *Journal Orofacial Pain*, **13**: 155–63.

Schindler, H.J., Svensson, P. (2007). Myofascial temporomandibular disorder pain. Pathophysiology and management. In: J.C. Turp, C., Sommer, A., Hugger (eds) *The Puzzle of Orofacial Pain. Integrating research into clinical management*, pp. 91–123. Karger, Basel.

Sessle, B.J. (1999). The neural basis of temporomandibular joint and masticatory muscle pain. *Journal Orofacial Pain*, **15**: 238–45.

Steenks, M.H., Hugger, A., de Wijer, A. (2007). Painful arthrogenous temporomandibular disorders. Pathophysiology, diagnosis and management. In: J.C.Turp, C. Sommer, A. Hugger (eds) *The Puzzle of Orofacial Pain. Integrating research into clinical management*, pp. 124–52. Karger, Basel.

Chapter 10

Trigeminal neuralgia

Joanna M. Zakrzewska and Mark E. Linskey

Key points

- Comprehensive history and examination including baseline measure of pain and quality of life essential
- MRI for diagnosis of symptomatic TN and evaluation of neurovascular compression
- Medical management starts with carbamazepine then trial of other drugs
- Refer early for a neurosurgical opinion
- Ablative surgery results in some degree of trigeminal nerve injury and gives pain relief for 3–5 years. Microvascular decompression offers longest pain free period with little sensory loss but risk of mortality
- Psychological support is important and need to provide access to written information
- Provide details of patient support group.

10.1 Chapter plan

Figure 10.1 is an outline of the main contents of this chapter.

10.2 Definition

Trigeminal neuralgia, a neuropathic pain, is defined by The International Association for the Study of Pain (ISAP) as 'a sudden and usually unilateral severe brief stabbing recurrent pain in the distribution of one or more branches of the fifth cranial nerve'.

Trigeminal neuralgia is classified as:

- idiopathic
- secondary – due to intrinsic brainstem pathology with trigeminal nerve, nuclei or tract involvement (e.g. multiple sclerosis or lacunar infarction), or due to extrinsic cerebellopontine angle pathology (e.g. neoplasms, benign or malignant or non-neoplastic cysts such as epidermoid, dermoid, or arachnoid cysts or vascular lesions such as aneurysms or arterio-venous malformations.)

Figure 10.1 Chapter plan

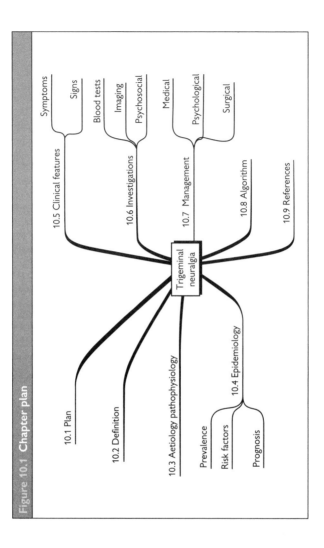

10.3 **Aetiology and pathophysiology**

Considerable progress has been made in elucidating the aetiology of this condition. In the majority of patients with classical trigeminal neuralgia the pain is generated due to compression of the trigeminal nerve most commonly at the root entry zone (point at which the peripheral and central myelin of the Schwann cells and oligodendrocutes, respectively, meet). The plaques of demyelination which occur lead to hyper-excitability of injured afferents which results in after discharges large enough to result in a non nociceptive signal being perceived as pain. The currently most widely accepted theory to explain trigeminal neuralgia is the one proposed by Devor and has been called the 'ignition theory'. It is likely that both central and peripheral changes occur which would account for why not all patients with a treated compression of the nerve get permanent relief. There are likely to be other factors involved given the rarity of the disease, and there may also be genetic causes.

10.4 **Epidemiology**

10.4.1 **Prevalence/incidence**
Trigeminal neuralgia is considered a rare condition with:
- crude annual incidence of 5.7 for women and 2.5 for men per 100,000
- peak incidence in the 50 to the 60 age group increasing with age
- point prevalence of 0.001.

A recent study using general practice research databases in the UK and very broad diagnostic criteria that may have allowed inclusion of neuropathic facial pain syndrome other than trigeminal neuralgia suggested a higher prevalence of 26.4 per 100,000.

10.4.2 **Risk factors**
The major risk factor is multiple sclerosis and hypertension may play a role but this is common in the age group at risk. Familial tendency is rare but possible. Bilateral involvement is present in only 6% of cases and sensory deficits are usually subtle and partial and are associated with either chronicity of the syndrome and/or a history of prior surgical intervention. Early, significant, as well as non-surgical sensory loss, in addition to bilateral involvement, should trigger a thorough investigation for symptomatic (i.e. secondary) trigeminal neuralgia.

10.4.3 **Prognosis**
Untreated the condition becomes gradually more severe with fewer remission periods but the rate at which this occurs is unpredictable at present. Spontaneous remission periods of up to 6 months are common, yet the syndrome remains predominantly progressive in nature. Up to 44% of patients

when followed for up to 16 years will fail to get complete pain relief with medical therapy. There is also data to suggest that the results of surgical intervention with microvascular decompression may begin to worsen if the syndrome has been allowed to persist for more than 8 years.

10.5 **Clinical features**

10.5.1 **Symptoms**

Classical trigeminal neuralgia is easily diagnosed and its diagnostic criteria have been described in the International Classification of Headache Disorders, although these criteria have not been validated. The most problematic feature of the diagnostic criteria is a requirement for absence of sensory deficit in the absence of prior surgical intervention history. There is abundant evidence that subtle clinically detectable sensory deficits are present in the setting of typical trigeminal neuralgia as well as evidence that electrophysiological abnormalities may antedate detectable sensory loss on examination. There are other forms of trigeminal neuralgia which most frequently have been called atypical trigeminal neuralgia and trigeminal neuropathy. As there are no long term cohort studies it is not possible to determine whether these atypical forms are in fact the same condition but further on in the natural history or whether they may represent a different pathophysiology.

The symptoms and signs of classical trigeminal neuralgia are summarized in Figure 10.2.

The timing of the attacks and remission periods as well as the character of the pain are the distinguishing features for classical trigeminal neuralgia. Many patients with trigeminal neuralgia report the severity of their pain being worse during the day and only a third of patients will report getting pain at night and result in awakening. Patients with other forms will describe a burning, dull aching after pain that is persistent and there is no completely pain-free interval.

Quality of life is severely impaired more so if the attacks are spontaneous as they reduce the ability to socialize as they are often provoked when eating and talking. Depression is common and suicides have been reported.

Many patients with trigeminal neuralgia will report a memorable onset and neurosurgeons have gone so far to suggest that this could be a prognostic factor for improved outcomes.

10.5.2 **Signs**

Although on routine examination most patients have no sensory deficit these may be very subtle and may increase in frequency with chronicity of the syndrome. Abnormalities in neurophysiological testing may identify subclinical deficits. Sensory testing is essential as this will potentially differentiate between symptomatic and idiopathic trigeminal neuralgia. Patients will exhibit tactile trigger areas within the trigeminal distribution which will precipitate an attack when stimulated. There are no autonomic features.

Figure 10.2 Major clinical features of trigeminal neuralgia

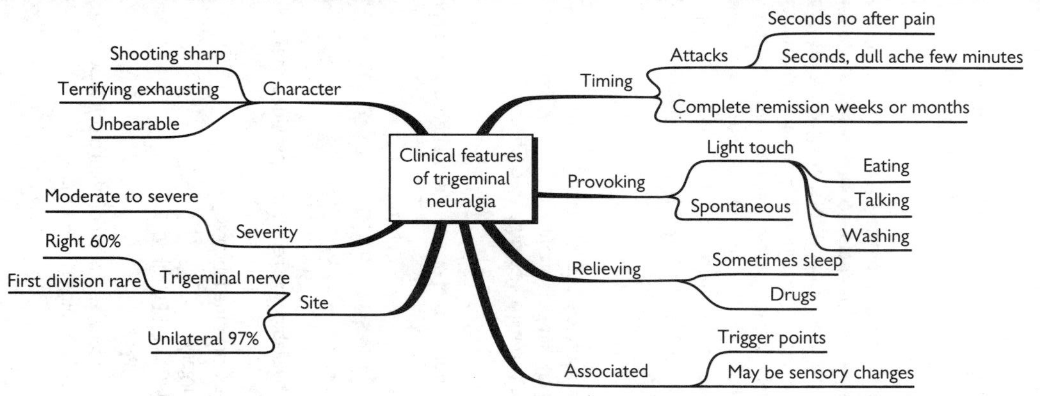

10.6 **Investigations**

10.6.1 **Blood tests**

None are required for diagnosis but basic haematological and biochemical investigations are important in monitoring patients on drug therapy.

10.6.2 **Imaging**

Radiological investigations are important to differentiate between symptomatic and idiopathic trigeminal neuralgia. MRI is useful to rule out secondary trigeminal neuralgia (e.g. neoplasms, cysts, aneurysms, AVM's, multiple sclerosis plaques and lacunar infarctions in the appropriate location). MRI can also detect compression from a dolichoectatic vertebrobasilar system which is useful for pre-operative counselling since this situation caries a higher risk of cranial nerve complication with subsequent microvascular decompression. MRI does not have sufficient positive- or negative predictive value to assess vascular compression as an etiology for the syndrome.

10.6.3 **Physiological**

Sensory testing is not done routinely but quantitative sensory testing QST's and evoked potentials may play an important role in differentiating between symptomatic and idiopathic trigeminal neuralgia (see Chapter 3 for more detail).

10.6.4 **Psychological**

These have been rarely reported but quality life is altered and depression is common pre-operatively.

10.7 **Management**

The following evidence is available and references provided at the end of the chapter:
- systematic reviews in the Cochrane Library
- systematic reviews on surgery
- regularly updated review Clinical Evidence
- PROGIDY guidelines for GPs
- Recommendations of European Federation of Neurological Societies (EFNS) and American Academy of Neurologists (AAN).

10.7.1 **Medical**

All patients will initially be treated medically and the commonly used drugs and the evidence for their use are shown in Table 10.1.

Table 10.1 Medical management of trigeminal neuralgia

Drug/therapy	Daily dose range	Efficacy NNT	Side effects	Comments
Proven in RCTs and effective				
Baclofen	50–80 mg	NNT 1.4 (1–2.6) only 10 patients, possibly effective	Ataxia, lethargy, fatigue, nausea, vomiting beware rapid withdrawal	Useful as add on therapy
Carbamazepine	300–1000 mg	NNT 2.6 (2–4), effective	Drowsiness, ataxia, headaches, nausea, vomiting constipation, blurred vision, rash, introduce slowly, drug interactions NNH 3.4 (2.5–5.2) for side effects, NNH for withdrawal 24 (13–110)	Reduced white cell count, hyponatrae-mia higher doses
Lamotrigine	200–400 mg	NNT 2.1 (1.3–6.1) as add on medication	Dizziness, drowsiness, constipation, ataxia, diplopia, irritability, rapid dose escalation leads to rashes	
Oxcarbazepine	300–1200 mg	effective	Vertigo, fatigue, dizziness, nausea, hyponatraemia in high doses, no major drug interactions	RCT only abstract cannot calculate NNT
Commonly used but no RCT				
Clonazepam	4–8 mg	low	Severe drowsiness – 60%, addictive	
Gabapentin	1800–3600 mg	good	Ataxia, dizziness, drowsiness, nausea, headache	Better tolerated than carbamaze-pine
Phenytoin	200–300 mg	good	Ataxia, lethargy, nausea, headache, behavioural changes, folate deficiency in prolonged use, gingival hypertrophy	Small margin for dose escalation, used intravenously for immediate effect
Pregabalin	150–600 mg	good	Ataxia, dizziness, drowsiness, nausea, headache	Rapid escalation possible
Valproic acid	600–1200 mg	poor	Irritability, restlessness, tremor, confusion, nausea, rash, weight gain	

Patients should keep pain diaries and change their drug levels to adjust to the changing severity of the pain and tolerability of side effects. Most of the drugs need to be escalated and withdrawn slowly to avoid side effects.

10.7.1.1 *Drugs used in RCTs*

These are or may be beneficial:

- Carbamazepine with good evidence to show that this drug is highly effective
- Oxcabazepine, daughter drug of carbamazepine, has been evaluated in RCTs and a small systematic review (all abstracts) comparing it to carbamazepine has been done. Although it is of similar efficacy to carbamazepine it is much better tolerated and results in fewer drug interactions. Long term follow has also shown that the drug is safe in long term use but that the pain gradually increases in severity and so the drug looses efficacy.
- Baclofen may be beneficial
- Lamotrigine as add on therapy may be beneficial

Ineffectiveness or the side effects profile are severe enough to exclude their use:

- Tocainide
- Tizanidine
- Pimozide
- Streptomycin injections at trigger points.

10.7.1.2 *Other drugs*

Pregabalin has been licensed for use in neuropathic pain and has been reported to be effective in a cohort series in trigeminal neuralgia. A recent randomized controlled trial suggests that gabapentin combined with repeated topical injections of ropivacain gives better pain control than gabapentin on its own. Clonazepam, valproate and phenytoin are often used.

There are no high quality studies on the use of polypharmacy as often practised in epilepsy.

Topical injections of lidocaine into trigger points can give some temporary relief.

10.7.2 **Psychological/non medical**

The fear, loneliness and depression associated with trigeminal neuralgia has been shown in data that patients have contributed to in the book on trigeminal neuralgia 'Insights – facts and stories behind trigeminal neuralgia'. Support groups can help to ease these feelings especially in reducing the isolation feelings and can also provide high quality patient friendly information.

National support groups have formed in many countries, e.g. US, UK, Australia, Germany and they provide some or all of the following:

- Books
- Leaflets
- Internet information http://www.tna-support.org/, http://www.tna.org, http://www.tna.org.uk/, http://www.stemer.de, http://www.tnaaustralia.org.au
- Email and chat rooms

- Phone lines
- Conferences with healthcare professionals.

10.7.3 **Surgical**

A decision analysis study using 156 patients with trigeminal neuralgia showed that they preferred surgical management to medical. However the timing of this decision has not been determined. Of the surgical procedures, there is a very slight preference for microvascular decompression.

There is insufficient evidence to determine which is the most successful surgical treatment as there are no RCTs of the major surgical procedures. In view of the lack of RCTs only those studies which have used independent observers to assess outcomes have been used to provide evidence. These are summarized in Table 10.2.

127

Table 10.2 Surgical management of trigeminal neuralgia*

Procedure	% Probability of being pain free	Mortality	Morbidity
Peripheral – neurectomy, cryotherapy, alcohol, injection, acupuncture	Two years – 22	Nil	Low, sensory loss, transient heamatoma, oedema
Radiofrequency thermorhizotomy (RFT)	Two years – 68 Five years – 48	Low	complications mainly relating to trigeminal nerve, dyseasthesia, anesthesia dolorosa, eye problems, masticatory problems, sensory loss over 50%
Percutaneous glycerol rhizotomy	Two years – 63 Five years – 45	Low	complications as for RFT but fewer cases of sensory loss
Balloon microcompression	Two years –79	Low	complications as for RFT, fewer with sensory loss but temporary masticatory problems common
Microvascular decompression	Two years – 81 Five years – 76 Ten years – 70	0.4%	Overall 75% no complications, 16% peri-operative complications, 2% transient cranial nerve 4th, 6th, 4% 8th dysfunction with 2 % permanent deafness
Gamma Knife surgery	Two years – 58	Nil	Late onset of relief, may only be partial, 7% sensory loss up to two years post treatment
* Data on 5 years not available for some procedures			

Surgical management can be carried out at three different levels:

- Peripheral at trigger points, e.g. cryotherapy, laser-therapy, alcohol injections and neurectomies.
- Gasserian ganglion level – all of which are ablative, radiofrequency thermocoagulation, percutaneous glycerol rhizotomy, balloon microcompression, and stereotactic radiosurgery (including Gamma Knife)
- Posterior fossa nerve root procedures – ablative partial sensory rhizotomy or stereotactic radiosurgery (including Gamma Knife) or non destructive – microvascular decompression.

10.7.4 **Peripheral procedures**

These are done under local anaesthesia and have few side effects. All provide only short term pain relief mostly under one year. Topical corneal lidocaine for V1 division trigeminal neuralgia has been assessed in RCT with a null result.

10.7.5 **Gasserian ganglion procedures**

These ablative procedures aim to reduce sensory transmission and hence pain. A needle is passed through the foramen ovale under radiographic control using either heavy sedation or light general anesthetic as shown in Figure 10.3.

Once within the ganglion one of three procedures can be carried out:

- Radio-frequency thermocoagulation – the nerve is damaged by temperatures between 60 and 90°C
- Percutaneous glycerol rhizotomy – the nerve is bathed in glycerol
- Balloon microcompression – the nerve is compressed by a Foley catheter balloon.
- stereotactic radiosurgery – the ganglion is irradiated with a single highly focussed and high dose of ionizing radiation

Patients are usually treated as outpatients but occasionally an overnight stay in hospital is required.

The results are fairly similar and the median pain relief period is 4 to 5 years. Complications will include:

- Varying degrees of sensory deficit including anesthesia dolorosa
- Other trigeminal nerve injuries such as masticatory problems
- Arrhythmias, aseptic meningitis and temporary diplopia in balloon compressions.

10.7.6 **Posterior fossa procedures**

The procedures done at this level include:

- Stereotactic radiosurgery, e.g. Gamma knife
- Partial sensory rhizotomy – this is done if no compression of the nerve is found
- Microvascular decompression.

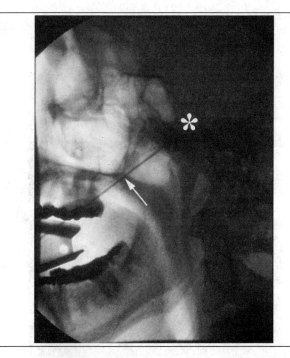

Figure 10.3 Percutaneous glycerol rhizotomy. Lateral intraoperative fluoroscopic view of a needle being passed through the cheek outside the mouth through the opening in the skull base for the trigeminal nerve (foramen ovale) to reach the ganglion of the nerve during a chemical glycerol rhizotomy. Arrow indicates position of needle, star ganglion.

The first two are ablative procedures and thus risk sensory loss. Stereotactic radiosurgery consists of delivering a high dose of irradiation, usually 70 to 90 Gy, to a small area (isocentre) of the cisternal portion of the trigeminal nerve. The procedure is carried out under local anaesthesia with light sedation and patients can be discharged within 24 hours. MRI sequencing is performed in order to identify the trigeminal nerve in its course from the pons into the Gasserian ganglion. See Figure 10.4 for location of dose.

In patients with pacemakers or who are treated with technologies requiring CT targeting, intrathecal CT cisternography with iodine dye injected in the CSF is utilized to visualize and target the trigeminal nerve root.

Stereotactic radiosurgery is the safest of all ablative techniques. Pain relief is similar to that of other ablative procedures but only 10% of patients report some form of sensory loss and in a very small group it can be severe. On the other hand, stereotactic radiosurgery is the only ablative procedure that does not produce immediate pain relief, usually requiring a median of 3–6 weeks for therapeutic effect.

Figure 10.4 A & B microvascular decompression

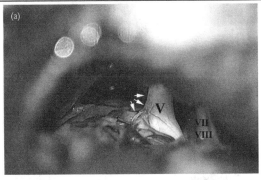

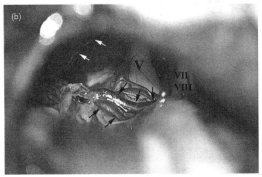

Intraoperative photographs under the operating microscope in a patient with right-sided TN showing the trigeminal nerve (V) and the seventh and eighth nerve complex (VII & VIII). The trigeminal nerve is compressed from below by a loop of the superior cerebellar artery (white arrow heads in figures A & B). Once the artery is moved away and the ala of the cerebellum mobilized to show where the nerve tangentially blends with the brain stem (figure B), the nerve is also found to be cross compressed from above by two veins (black arrow heads).

Microvascular decompression is an open micro-neurosurgical procedure that involves entry into the posterior fossa, identification of the vascular compression and dislodging the vessel/s from the trigeminal nerve. See Figure 10.5 for examples.

This can be achieved either by the use of shredded Teflon felt or by making vascular slings to keep the offending vessels away from the nerve.

If no compression is found then some surgeons consider sectioning part of the sensory nerve. The rate of 'negative explorations' tends to reflect ongoing disagreement among surgeons as to whether arteries are indenting the nerve or just touching the nerve, and whether or not compressing small artery branches or even veins should be considered clinically significant. In Jannetta's series and those of his trainees, negative explorations are encountered in <5% of patients with the classical clinical syndrome.

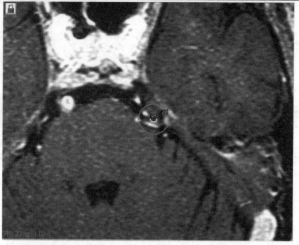

Figure 10.5 Targeting MR scan for Gamma surgery showing the radiation focus spot targeted on the trigeminal nerve root

The inner line is the 95% dose prescription line and the outer line shows the limit for 20% of the prescription dose. The brainstem receives less than 20% of the prescription dose.

After microvascular decompression, 80% of patients are initially pain-free with no medication requirements. At 10–20 years 70% of patients may still remain pain free. Most recurrences occur within the first 2 years.

As this is a major surgical procedure it results in early complications:

- 0.4% mortality
- cerebral infarcts and haemorrhage resulting in strokes (<2%)
- meningitis both bacterial and aseptic (<5%)
- CFS leaks (<5%).

As well as complications common to all instances of general anesthesia and hospitalization:

- Pulmonary emboli (<1%)
- Gastro-intestinal bleeds (<1%).

The major long term neurological deficit is that of an ipsilateral hearing loss. Ipsilateral deafness occurs in 1–2% of patients, but this incidence is doubled if intraoperative auditory brain stem evoked response monitoring is not utilized. Sensory loss is often present in those who undergo partial sensory rhizotomy but can also occur after microvascular decompression. An independent satisfaction survey has shown up to 75% are satisfied with their outcomes and the majority would have preferred to have the procedure earlier.

In those patients who do not want to undergo major surgery or are not fit for it then the ablative procedures at the Gasserian ganglion level can lead to acceptable pain relief and freedom from the need to use drugs. Gamma knife procedures are the least invasive but there is least long term data.

There is no quality evidence to provide guidance on management of patients with multiple sclerosis or those who undergo a recurrence of pain.

10.8 **Algorithm**

The algorithm below provides a possible evidence based approach to management of trigeminal neuralgia – Figure 10.6.

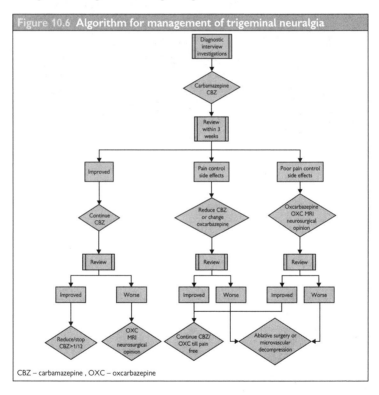

Figure 10.6 Algorithm for management of trigeminal neuralgia

CBZ – carbamazepine , OXC – oxcarbazepine

Anonymous. (2004). The International Classification of Headache Disorders: 2nd edition. *Cephalalgia*, **24**: Suppl 1, 9–160.

Cruccu, G., Gronseth, G., Alksne, J., Argoff, C., Burchiel, K., Nurmikko, T.J. and Zakrzewska, J. AAN-EFNS Guidelines on management of trigeminal neuralgia. (2008). *European Journal of Neurology*, 1468–1331. In press.

Devor, M., Amir, R. and Rappaport, Z.H. (2002). Pathophysiology of trigeminal neuralgia: the ignition hypothesis. *Clinical Journal of Pain*, **18**: 4–13.

He, L., Wu, B. and Zhou, M. (2006). Non-antiepileptic drugs for trigeminal neuralgia. *Cochrane Database of Systematic Reviews*, **3**: CD004029.

Lopez, B.C., Hamlyn, P.J. and Zakrzewska, J.M. (2004). Systematic review of ablative neurosurgical techniques for the treatment of trigeminal neuralgia. *Neurosurgery*, **54**: 973–82.

Merskey, H. and Bogduk, N. (1994). *Classification of Chronic Pain. Descriptors of chronic pain syndromes and definitions of pain terms*, 2nd edn, pp. 1–222. IASP Press, Seattle.

Nurmikko, T.J. and Eldridge, P.R. (2001). Trigeminal neuralgia – pathophysiology, diagnosis and current treatment. *British Journal of Anaesthesia*, **87**: 117–32.

Spatz, A.L., Zakrzewska, J.M. and Kay, E.J. (2007). Decision analysis of medical and surgical treatments for trigeminal neuralgia: How patient evaluations of benefits and risks affect the utility of treatment decisions. *Pain*, **131**: 302–10.

Weigel, G. and Casey, K.F. (2004). *Striking Back: The Trigeminal Neuralgia and Face Pain Handbook.*, The Trigeminal Neuralgia Association. Gainesville, Florida, USA.

Wiffen, P.J., Collins, S., McQuay, H., Carroll, D., Jadad, A. and Moore, A. (2005a). Anticonvulsant drugs for acute and chronic pain. *Cochrane Database Systematic Reviews* CD001133.

Wiffen, P.J., McQuay, H.J. and Moore, R.A. (2005b). Carbamazepine for acute and chronic pain. *Cochrane Database Systematic Reviews* CD005451.

Zakrzewska, J.M. (2006). *Insights: facts and stories behind trigeminal neuralgia*, pp. 1–403. Trigeminal Neuralgia Association, Gainesville, Florida, USA.

Zakrzewska, J.M. and Lopez, B.C. (2006). Trigeminal neuralgia. *BMJ Clinical Evidence Concise*, 462–4. See also http://www.clinicalevidence.com.

Website: PROGIDY guidelines http://www.cks.library.nhs.uk/

Chapter 11

Neuropathic pain

Suthipun Jitpimolmard and Steven Graff Radford

Key points

- Trigeminal neuropathic pain is due to trauma to the trigeminal nerve and may be the same as atypical odontalgia
- Trigeminal post herpetic neuralgia has the same features and management as postherpetic neuralgia elsewhere in the body
- Glossopharyngeal neuralgia is much rarer than trigeminal neuralgia and its management is largely the same
- Giant cell arteritis results in unilateral most commonly temporal pain that must be recognised rapidly as steroids will prevent the occurrence of blindness
- Migraines are common unilateral headaches that often co-exist with facial pain
- Acute treatment as well as prophylaxis is available for migraineurs who tend to improve with age
- Tension type headaches often co-exist with facial pain and need to be managed with medical and behavioural methods.

11.1 Chapter plan

Figure 11.1 is an outline of the main contents of this chapter. The chapter describes a variety of conditions classified as neuropathic pains and primary headaches which have not been described in other chapters – Chapter 7, 8, 10 and 12. Only the most common will be described and other more detailed texts should be consulted for the rare causes of trigeminal neurovascular pains.

11.2 Traumatic induced neuralgia or trigeminal neuropathic pain

11.2.1 Definition

This is a condition in which trauma has occurred to the trigeminal nerve, which can vary in its extent from a single nerve to the whole face, and has then

Figure 11.1 **Chapter plan**

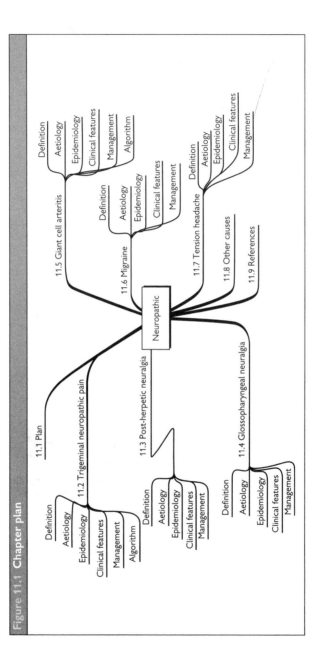

Figure 11.1 **Chapter plan**

Neuropathic

11.1 Plan

11.2 Trigeminal neuropathic pain
- Definition
- Aetiology
- Epidemiology
- Clinical features
- Management
- Algorithm

11.3 Post-herpetic neuralgia
- Definition
- Aetiology
- Epidemiology
- Clinical features
- Management

11.4 Glossopharyngeal neuralgia
- Definition
- Aetiology
- Epidemiology
- Clinical features
- Management

11.5 Giant cell arteritis
- Definition
- Aetiology
- Epidemiology
- Clinical features
- Management
- Algorithm

11.6 Migraine
- Definition
- Aetiology
- Epidemiology
- Clinical features
- Management

11.7 Tension headache
- Definition
- Aetiology
- Epidemiology
- Clinical features
- Management

11.8 Other causes

11.9 References

resulted in pain and or changes in sensation. This disorder is also called deafferentation, dysesthesia and often relegated to the old category of atypical facial pain or if very localized termed atypical odontalgia (see Chapter 8). It may in time be that in future this terminology will be used instead of atypical odontalgia. It is also sometimes called trigeminal neuropathy.

11.2.2 **Aetiology and Pathophysiology**

There are a number of mechanisms that can cause traumatic induced neuropathy. They can be described as:

- Peripheral sensitization
- Ectopic activity due to sodium channel expression
- Central sensitization
- Beta fibre reorganization
- Alteration in central inhibition systems
- Sympathetically maintained pain due to alpha receptor sprouting.

More than one mechanism may be involved.

11.2.3 **Epidemiology**

Currently there is no data on this specific condition. It has been suggested that a risk factor could be lack of adequate anesthesia for dental procedures.

11.2.4 **Clinical Features**

There are still no case controlled studies describing the diagnostic criteria and the International Headache Society classification (IHS) does not provide any criteria. The pain is described as a continuous burning sensation localized to the area that has been injured. The neuranatomical distribution of the pain will vary greatly depending on the extent of trauma – very local if related to a single tooth or extensive if related to facial trauma. The nerve dysfunction can manifest itself as a negative symptom, i.e. sensory loss or as a positive one in the form of allodynia, hyperalgesia, and parasthesia and these can be detected on examination. Careful dental examination and assessment of temporomandibular muscular should be included as well as careful neurological examination. The clinical features are shown in Figure 11.2.

1.2.5 **Investigations**

Imaging is done to rule out central processes such as tumour, vascular compression and infection.

Local inspection and evaluation should include a detailed neurological screening assessing for sensory change, allodynia, hyperalgesia and other sensory changes such as described in Chapter 3 section 3.2. A recent publication has shown that these patients all have abnormal qualitative sensory changes whereas those called atypical facial pain are less likely to be positive for all tests. Neural blockade either sensory or sympathetic may help define the pathophysiology.

Figure 11.2 Clinical features of trigeminal neuropathic pain

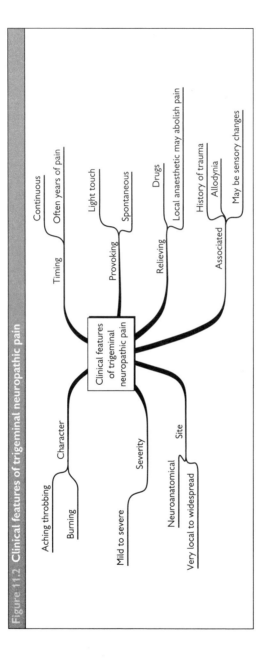

Attempts have been made to prepare self complete questionnaires to help diagnosis neuropathic pain and there are now several of these in use and discussed in another book in the series – 'Neuropathic Pain', see references.

11.2.6 **Management**

Management may require a number of interventions. There are no specific RCTS for trigeminal neuropathic pain and most of the data is extrapolated from general guidelines on neuropathic pain, including post herpetic neuralgia, which are covered in the volume on neuropathic pain and shown in Table 11.1.

Table 11.1 Treatment of trigeminal neuropathic pain and post herpetic neuralgia. There are no trials in trigeminal neuropathic pain specifically

Drug/therapy	Daily dose range	Efficacy NNT very good, good, low	Side effects NNH	Comments
Proven in RCTs				
Nortriptyline	25–100 mg	NNT 3.6	NNH 6, sedation, dry mouth, weight gain	Use 6–8 weeks at least, 2 at max tolerated dose
Venlafaxine	37.5–225 mg	NNT 3.1	NNH 9.6 nausea	Use at least 4–6 weeks
Duloxetine	30–120 mg	good	Nausea	Use 4 weeks
Gabapentin	100–3600 mg	good	Sedation, dizziness, peripheral oedema	Use at least 10 weeks with slow titration
Pregabalin	150–600 mg	good	Sedation, dizziness, peripheral oedema	Use 4 weeks
Lidocaine 5% patch	3 patches max	good	Local erythema, rash	Use 3 weeks
Morphine, oxycodone, methadone	10–15 mg four hourly	low	Nausea, constipation, drowsiness, addiction	Monitor by specialist
Tramadol	100–400 mg daily	NNT 3.8	NNH 8.3 constipation, nausea, sedation	4 weeks

NNT Number needed to treat, NNH number needed to harm.

Many of these drugs should be titrated up slowly over a few weeks and maximum doses do not need to be used.

11.2.6.1 *Pharmacologic interventions*

- Tricyclic antidepressants especially nortriptyline
- Selective serotonin, norepinepherine reuptake inhibitors
- Antiepileptic drugs particularly the calcium channel ligands such as gabapentin and pregabalin
- Analgesics.

11.2.6.2 *Topical therapy*

Topical anaesthetic, or other medications such as capsaicin, amitriptyline, ketoprofen or carbamazepine may be delivered to the injured site with the aid of a neurosensory shield or stent. The stent or small splint if intra-oral is fashioned from acrylic and made to cover the painful site. The patient wears it at all times applying the topical agent intermittently.

11.2.6.3 *Surgical intervention*

There are case series reporting the following procedures but there is no good quality evidence for these:

- Repeated neural blockade (sympathetic)
- Sympathetic radiofrequency
- Gamma knife to the sphenopalatine ganglion
- Brain stimulation.

Nerve repair can also be attempted and this is done for nerves damaged during oral surgical procedures and can be helpful especially if the repair is done early.

11.2.6.4 *Psychological*

As detailed in Chapter 5 section 5.5 this will be helpful.

11.2.6.5 *Other therapies*

Acupuncture and TENS.

11.2.7 **Algorithm**

Figure 11.3 suggests an algorithm for treatment of trigeminal neuropathic pain.

11.3 Post-herpetic neuralgia (PHN)

11.3.1 **Definition**

The presence of persistent burning pain accompanied by intermittent shooting sensation localized to the site of previous herpes zoster infection. By definition post-herpetic neuralgia (PHN) occurs 3–6 months after the infection has cleared.

11.3.2 **Aetiology and Pathophysiology**

The cause of PHN is the herpes zoster virus. Once exposed, usually from chicken pox, the virus lies dormant in the ganglion and when activated causes the classic rash of herpes zoster. The virus results in damage to the nerve and produces PHN.

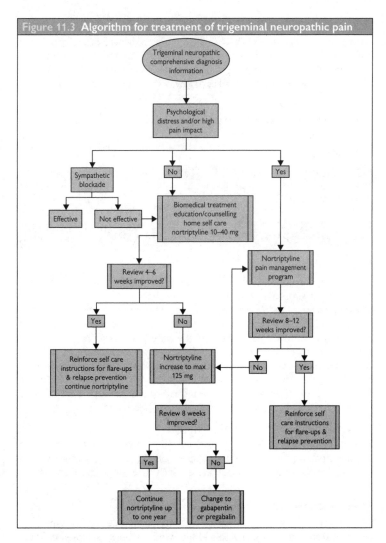

Figure 11.3 Algorithm for treatment of trigeminal neuropathic pain

11.3.3 **Epidemiology**

PHN occurs in 40% of patients who have herpes zoster; the majority are over the age of 70 years. Patients who are immunocompromized are also more likely to develop herpes zoster.

11.3.4 **Clinical Features**

The clinical presentation of PHN is the same as anywhere in the rest of the body; it can present inside the mouth but is more frequently noted extraorally. The pain is a continuous burning pain punctuated by intermittent shooting pain. Allodynia and hyperalgesia, as well as patchy numbness are often noted.

11.3.5 **Investigations**

None are needed although sometimes there can be an underlying malignancy. If <50 may need to consider HIV infection.

11.3.6 **Management**

Aggressive therapy with antivirals in the acute zoster phase is essential. Once PHN has developed therapy is similar to that of traumatic neuralgia as described above and in Table 11.2.

11.4 **Glossopharyngeal neuralgia (GPN)**

11.4.1 **Definition**

The International Association for the Study of Pain (IASP) defines the condition as sudden, severe, brief, recurrent pains in the distribution of the glosso-pharyngeal nerve. The IHS recently classified GPN into classic and symptomatic. The classic GPN is a severe transient stabbing pain experienced in the ear, base of the tongue, tonsilar fossa or beneath the angle of the jaw. The pain is felt in the distributions of the auricular and pharyngeal branches of the vagus nerve and glossopharyngeal nerve. It is commonly provoked by swallowing, talking or coughing. It may remit for varying periods. Secondary GPN presents with the added presence of an aching pain that may persist between attacks and a causative lesion is demonstrated by special investigations or surgery.

11.4.2 **Aetiology and Pathophysiology**

The exact mechanism is not known but is probable that it is similar to trigeminal neuralgia in that there is compression of the nerve. Secondary GTN can be due to congenital abnormalities such as Arnold-Chiari as well as malignancies.

11.4.3 **Epidemiology**

GPN is very rare with an incidence rate of 0.7 per 100,000, six times less common than trigeminal neuralgia and the two conditions can co-exist. There slight predominance in women and patients over 50 years.

11.4.4 **Clinical Features**

These are the IHS Criteria for classical glossopharyngeal neuralgia:

(a) Paroxysmal attacks of facial pain lasting from a fraction of a second to 2 minutes and fulfilling criteria B and C.

(b) Pain has all of the following characteristics:

- unilateral location
- distribution within the posterior part of the tongue, tonsilar fossa, pharynx or beneath the angle of the lower jaw and / or in the ear.
- sharp, stabbing and severe
- precipitated by swallowing, chewing talking, coughing or yawning

(c) Attacks are stereotyped in the individual patient

(d) There is no clinically evident neurological deficit

(e) Not attributable to another disorder.

GPN occurs in episodes like trigeminal neuralgia (TN) with each episode lasting for weeks to months, but in some patients can be unremitting. GPN is almost always unilateral. The right side is affected more often with GPN than with TN. Bilateralism was noted less often in TN than in GPN cases. See Figure 11.4 for the clinical features.

11.4.5 **Investigations**

Imaging to rule out central causes such as tumor, infection or vascular compression should include brain MRI. Further Eagle's Syndrome should be ruled out. This is due to elongation of the styloid process which can then press on glossopharyngeal, vagus, and/or trigeminal nerves. The pain associated with this condition is often unilateral and can occur in the throat and ear as in GPN.

11.4.6 **Management**

11.4.6.1 *Pharmacological*

There are no RCTS and so the treatments are the same as for trigeminal neuralgia (see Chapter 10). In patients who also present with cardiac syncope cardiac pacing may be required.

11.4.6.2 *Surgical*

Glossopharyngeal nerve decompression appears to provide the best outcome but there are very few studies.

Glossopharyngeal nerve neurectomy has been reported but the results are poor.

11.4.7 **Algorithm**

This is similar to trigeminal neuralgia (see Figure 10.6 in Chapter 10) but there is less quality evidence.

11.5 **Giant cell arteritis (GCA)**

11.5.1 **Definition**

Giant cell arteritis (GCA) is defined as 'unilateral or bilateral headache, mainly continuous with aching or throbbing pain, sometimes very intense, usually in the elderly, with signs of temporal artery' with pathonogmonic histological

Figure 11.4 The clinical features of glossopharyngeal neuralgia

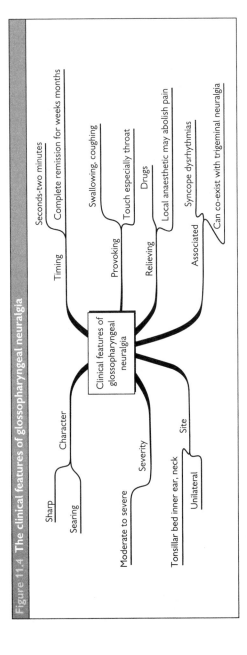

appearance of mononucleated giant cells in the blood vessel. The condition is not confined to this anatomical location. GCA is also known by different names including Horton's arteritis and temporal arteritis.

11.5.2 **Aetiology and Pathophysiology**

This disorder is caused by cell mediated immune damage which results in an intense active inflammatory response. It would appear that the primary antigen is elastin but what the actual trigger is remains unknown. Vessels particularly affected are the head arteries, mostly branches of the external carotid artery.

11.5.3 **Epidemiology**

There appears to be a geographic variation in the incidence with the highest numbers being recorded in the Nordic races. This suggests there may be a genetic predisposition. Long term prognosis is good but relapses occur and these may continue for many years. Up to a third of patients may die and this was more likely to happen in those who become permanently blind or who need larger doses of steroids to control their symptoms.

11.5.4 **Clinical Features**

The IHS lists the criteria as:

(a) Any new persisting headache

(b) At least one of the following:
- Swollen tender scalp-artery with elevated erythrocyte sedimentation rate (ESR) or C reactive protein (CRP)
- Temporal artery biopsy demonstrating giant cell arteritis

(c) Headache occurs in close temporal relation to other symptoms of giant cell arteritis

(d) Major improvement or disappearance of headache within 3 days of high dose steroid treatment.

Of all arteritis and collagen vascular diseases, GCA is the disease most conspicuously associated with headache.

The clinical features are shown in Figure 11.5.

11.5.4.1 *Clinical symptoms*

The following points should be alerting signs for diagnosis of GCA:
- Recent persisting headache occurring in people over 60 years
- The variability in the characteristics of headache
- Range of associated symptoms e.g. polymyalgia rheumatica, jaw claudication, generalized changes upset such as weight loss, neurological changes such as ataxia, numbness
  Recent repeated attacks of loss of vision.

Figure 11.5 The clinical features of giant cranial arteritis

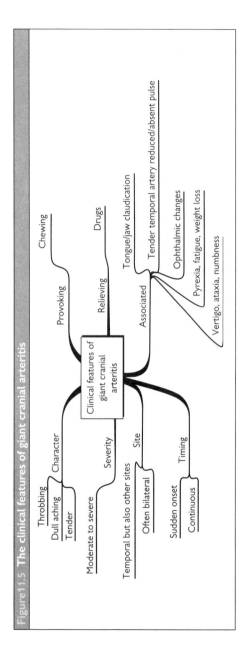

11.5.4.2 *Clinical signs*

These may show any or all of these features:

- Tender scalp arteries with reduced or absent pulses
- Ophthalmic changes including: Visual field constriction, visual loss, optic atrophy, scleritis, episcleritis, proptosis, ptosis, diplopia
- Neurological changes such as posterior circulation stroke
- Limb ischaemia with possible tender limb arteries, bruits, pulse asymmetry
- Congestive cardiac failure.

The time interval between visual loss in one eye and in the other is usually less than 1 week. The major risk is that of blindness due to anterior ischemic optic neuropathy. There is also a risk of cerebral ischemic events and of dementia.

11.5.5 **Investigations**

11.5.5.1 *Blood tests*

All patients over the age of 50 with unilateral headache should have an erythrocyte sedimentation rate (ESR) performed – a level over 50 mm/hour may be significant. ESR can be elevated by many infectious, inflammatory or rheumatic disorders and increases with age. A normal ESR rules out GCA but a high one does not rule it in. The C-reactive protein is markedly elevated – over 0.5 mg/dl. There may also be mild anaemia, thrombocytopaenia, elevated serum enzymes like aspartate transaminase and alkaline phosphatase.

11.5.5.2 *Imaging*

Duplex scanning of the temporal arteries may visualize the thickened arterial wall (as a halo on axial sections) and may help to select the site for biopsy.

11.5.5.3 *Histology*

At histology, the temporal artery may be uninvolved in some areas (skip areas) pointing to the necessity of serial sectioning and a 4–6 cm segment of temporal artery should be removed.

11.5.6 **Management**

Pharmacologic intervention with high dose steroid is usually successful. Intravenous methylprednisolone 0.5–1 mg/kg body weight is the starting dose and is then slowly reduced to around 40 mg/day within 4–6 weeks of initiating therapy. Rapid resolution of headache and constitutional symptoms within days is a good indicator that the diagnosis is correct. Reductions in steroid dosage can be made by 2.5–5 mg a day every 2–4 weeks and guided by the patient's symptoms and regular checking of the ESR.

This steroid can then be replaced by methotrexate at a weekly dose of 7.5–12.5 mg weekly with folic acid cover.

11.5.7 **Algorithm**

The algorithm for treatment is shown in Figure 11.6.

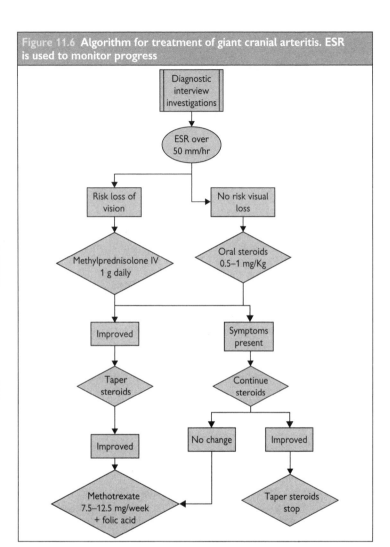

Figure 11.6 Algorithm for treatment of giant cranial arteritis. ESR is used to monitor progress

The next section will briefly describe the primary headaches as patients with orofacial pain often have headaches as co-morbid conditions and they need to be differentiated from other forms of pain in the first division of the trigeminal nerve. For more detail the neurology texts should be accessed. Table 11.2 compares and contrasts the features of these trigeminal neuropathic pains.

11.6 Migraine

11.6.1 Definition

Chronic headache disorder manifesting in attacks lasting 4–7 hours. The typical characteristics of headache are unilateral location, pulsating quality, moderate or severe intensity, aggravation by routine physical activity and association with nausea, photophobia and phonophobia.

Table 11.2 Clinical features of pains presenting principally in the first trigeminal division

	Migraine	Tension-type headache	Giant cell artertits
Site and radiation	unilateral fronto temporal	bilateral band around head	unilateral, temporal
Character	throbbing	achy, pressure	throbbing
Periodicity	intermittent	intermittent	continuous
Duration	4–72 hours	30 minutes – days	continuous
Severity	moderate to severe	mild to moderate	moderate to severe
Provoking factors	stress physical activity foods, odors, estrogen, alcohol, barometric pressure, sleep issues changes	stress, body postures	pressure over temporal artery
Relieving factors	medications sleep	medications exercise, stretching	medications
Associated factors	nausea, vomiting, photo and phonophobia	none	jaw claudication
Examination	neurological	neurological, muscle palpation, skeletal assessment	neurological, erythrocyte sedimentation rate, temporal artery biopsy

11.6.2 Aetiology and Pathophysiology

While there is usually a family history, the exact genetic link is not known. Migraine pathophysiology is best discussed using the four clinical stages (premonitory, aura, headache and recovery) as a guide.

Migraine aura is associated with cortical depolarization and spreading electrical activity, it is initiated following activation of a 'migraine generator' located in the midbrain. The pain is due to a neural inflammatory process in the meninges. Peptides released by trigeminal afferents create pain and cause secondary vasodilatation. Nociceptive input then travels to the trigeminal nucleus, thalamus and cortex.

11.6.3 **Epidemiology**

Migraine begins in childhood as early as it can be described and it is a common disease. There is an increase in frequency with the incidence comparable in males and females until puberty when there is an increased frequency seen in females, 17% of females and 6% of males. Migraine is unilateral in 60% of cases. The headaches peak in the 4th decade and then decline. It is being postulated that migraine may change with time and transform to one that is located more on the lower face and the term facial migraine may then be used.

11.6.4 **Clinical Features**

The IHS has defined migraine with the following features:

Diagnostic criteria:

A At least 5 attacks fulfilling B-D.

B Headache attacks lasting 4–72 hours (untreated or unsuccessfully treated)

C Headache has at least two of the following characteristics:

• Unilateral location

• Pulsating quality

• Moderate or severe pain intensity

• Aggravation by or causing avoidance from routine physical activity (i.e. walking or climbing stairs)

D During headache at least one of the following:

• Nausea and/or vomiting

• Photophobia and phonophobia

E Not attributed to another disorder

F Migraine aura occurs in approximately 15% of migraine patients, 10% of the time.

11.6.5 **Investigations**

There is no necessity to image the head in a patient who presents with a long history of unchanged migraine. Imaging is recommended in those patients who:

• Report a substantial change in headache pattern, associated with focal neurological symptoms

• The first headache ever, the worst headache ever or new onset headache in the elderly

• History of seizures

• Symptomatic illness such as acquired immunodeficiency syndrome, tumours, or neurofibromatosis.

The American Academy of Neurology has concluded that CT and MRI are not likely to significantly increase diagnostic yield or uncover pathologic entities.

11.6.6 **Management**

There are several Cochrane reviews on management of migraine as well as regularly updated topics in BMJ Clinical Evidence available on the internet.

11.6.6.1 *Pharmacological*

Table 11.3 summarizes therapies that are used for migraines.

Acute Therapy: The goals of acute therapy are to treat the pain as rapidly as possible, restoring function, minimizing recurrence or the need for backup medications while allowing the patients the feeling of self control. Frequent acute medication use (greater than two headache days per week on a regular basis) may result in rebound headache. Currently, there are various medications

Table 11.3 Acute therapies for migraine oral unless stated otherwise		
Drug	**Dose**	**Comment**
Non specific for which there is high level of recommendation		
Acetylsalicylic acid (ASA)	1000 mg/6h (PO)	Gastrointestinal, risk of bleeding
Ibuprofen	200–800 mg/8h	Gastrointestinal, risk of bleeding
Naproxen	500–1000 mg/day	Gastrointestinal, risk of bleeding
Diclofenac	50 mg/8h	Gastrointestinal, risk of bleeding
Paracetamol	1000 mg/6h	Care in liver and kidney failure
ASA plus, paracetamol plus caffeine	250 mg, 200–250 mg and 50 mg	Gastrointestinal, risk of bleeding care renal and kidney failure
Specific for which there is high level recommendation		
Sumatriptan	25, 50, 100 mg (PO), 25 mg (S), 10–20 mg (N) 6 mg (SC)	
Zolmitriptan	2.5–5 mg (PO), 2.5–5 mg (N)	
Naratriptan	2.5 mg	Less but longer efficacy than sumatriptan
Rizatriptan	10 mg	5 mg when taking propranolol
Almotriptan	12.5 mg	Probably less side effects than sumatriptan
Eletriptan	20 and 40 mg	Can use 80 mg if 40 mg not effective
Frovatriptan	2.5 mg	Less but longer efficacy than sumatriptan
Anti-emetic to combine with one from above		
Metoclopramide	10–20 mg (PO), 20 mg (S), 10 mg (IM,IV,S)	Side effect: dyskinesia; contraindicated in childhood and in pregnancy
Domperidon	20-30 mg	Side effects less severe than in metoclopramide
PO – oral, N – nasal, SC subcutaneous, IM intramuscular, IV intravenous, S suppository		

available, some specific and some not specific to migraine. Patients need to be provided some hierarchy and instructions on use and this can initially be done in primary care or if not successful in special headache clinics.

Prophylactic Therapy: The goals of migraine preventative therapy are to reduce attack frequency, severity and duration while improving response to acute therapy and restoring function.

Preventative therapy should be considered if:

• The migraines interfere with daily function
• More frequent than twice weekly
• Acute medications are insufficient or ineffective at controlling the headache
• Specific contraindication or acute medication overuse is occurring.

Prophylactic agents can be grouped into the following (expressed as total daily dose):

First line supported by good level of evidence

1. Beta Blockers – propranolol 40–240 mg, metoprolol 50–200 mg,
2. Calcium Channel Blockers – flunarizine 5–10 mg
3. Anti-Epileptic Agents – valproic acid 500–1800 mg, topiramate 25–100 mg

Evidence of efficacy, but less effective or more side effects than drugs 1–3.

4. Anti-depressants – amitriptyline 25–150 mg
5. Anti-Inflammatory Agents – naproxen 500–1000 mg

11.6.6.2 *Non pharmacologic therapy*

Patient education is a necessary and essential component to any treatment plan and should include a basic explanation of the headache as a physiological disorder.

Trigger factors are often discussed, although evidence is often only anecdotal and although the trigger factors are common to most people, each patient may experience their own unique list. Figure 11.7 shows the potential triggers.

11.6.6.3 *Psychological*

It is crucial to identify maladaptive thoughts, develop an action plan to deal with the headache and to encourage long term implementation of the techniques. Some of the techniques are covered in Chapter 5 section 5.5.

The following small placebo controlled trials of herbal therapies have shown possible benefits:

• Magnesium dicitrate 600 mg per day
• Riboflavin 400 mg per day
• Feverfew
• Petadolex.

11.6.6.4 *Physical modalities*

Botulinum toxin has been evaluated in 7 RCTs but the evidence for efficacy is conflicting. Other treatments that have been tried but not substantiated by high quality RCTs include: neural blockade , application of vapocoolant spray (Fluorimetnane), transcutaneous electrical stimulation TENS, acupuncture, intraoral splints, exercise, chiropractics, osteopathy, naturopathy, homeopathy.

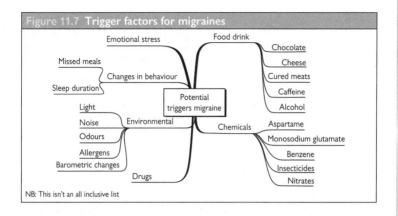

Figure 11.7 Trigger factors for migraines

Emotional stress

Food drink

Missed meals

Changes in behaviour

Sleep duration

Light

Noise

Odours

Allergens

Barometric changes

Environmental

Potential
triggers migraine

Chemicals

Drugs

Chocolate

Cheese

Cured meats

Caffeine

Alcohol

Aspartame

Monosodium glutamate

Benzene

Insecticides

Nitrates

NB: This isn't an all inclusive list

11.7 **Tension-type headache**

11.7.1 **Definition**
The IHS has divided tension-type headache into an episodic and a chronic form dependant on their frequency and presence of vomiting. The headaches are bilateral with a pressing quality of mild to moderate intensity and not aggravated by routine physical activity. There is no nausea or vomiting and low likelihood of photophobia or phonophobia.

11.7.2 **Aetiology and Pathophysiology**
The pathophysiology of tension-type headache is not understood. Most researchers believe that tension-type headache arises from local peripheral mechanisms, however some believe that there is a central mechanism to the pain.

11.7.3 **Epidemiology**
The overall prevalence of episodic tension-type headache in a population based study in a one year period was found to be 30–80%. Chronic tension type headache prevalence was 2.2% for the same year. Women had a higher prevalence then men for both types, male to female ratio of 1:1.3.

Prognosis is favorable with 45% being free of headaches by 3 years. About 16% remain chronic.

Risk factors for poor prognosis are chronic tension-type headache at baseline, coexisting migraine, single and sleep problems.

11.7.4 **Clinical features**
Episodic tension-type headache lasts from 30 minutes to 7 days, with a pressing or tightening (non-pulsatile) quality, of mild to moderate in intensity, bilateral in location, and not aggravated by routine physical activity such as walking a flight of stairs. There is no nausea or vomiting as is commonly associated with migraine. Also, photophobia or phonophobia, are not common, although one

may be present. Physical activity tends to reduce these headaches. Tension-type headaches can be localized to any part of the head, but are often described as a tight band around the head. The episodic form is defined by the IHS as having greater then ten lifetime attacks, but less then fifteen attacks per month. The chronic form occurs greater then fifteen times per month for at least 6 months. Chronic tension-type headache is not associated with vomiting as in the episodic form, but there can be one of the following: nausea, photophobia, or phonophobia. The presence of pericranial tenderness has been described as being associated with tension-type headache.

11.7.5 **Management**

There are several Cochrane reviews on management of tension (chronic) headaches as well as regularly updated topics in BMJ Clinical Evidence available on the internet.

A combination of medications or behavioral techniques are needed to enhance central inhibition while simultaneously reducing peripheral inputs through physical therapies.

11.7.5.1 *Pharmacological*

• Aspirin 500–1000 mg or other NSAIDs
• Simple analgesics with caffeine
• Preventive – amitriptyline 75–150 mg.

11.7.5.2 *Physical therapies*

• Specific stretching exercises aimed at improving body posture and mechanics
• Biofeedback
• Acupuncture may be helpful

11.8 **Other causes**

The following are some rare causes for facial pain which are not discussed as they need to be diagnosed by specialists but many of the diagnostic criteria can be found in the IHS classification.

• Tolosa-Hunt Syndrome
• Raeder's Syndrome
• Pre-trigeminal neuralgia
• Trigeminal neuropathy associated with connective tissue disorders
• Local and metastatic neoplasms
• Petrous apex infection/inflammation: Gradenigo's syndrome
• Cavernous sinus thrombosis or fistula
• Carotid artery dissection
• Intracranial aneurysms.

Anonymous. (2004). Classification and diagnostic criteria for headache disorders, cranial neuralgias and facial pain. Headache Classification Committee of the International Headache Society. *Cephalalgia*, **24** (Suppl 1).

Attal, N., Crucc G., Haanpää M., Hansson P., Jensen T.S., Nurmikko T., Sampaio C., Sindrup S., Wiffen P. (2006). EFNS Task Force. EFNS guidelines on pharmacological treatment of neuropathic pain. *European Journal Neurology*, **13**: 1153–69.

Bennett, M. (2006). *Neuropathic Pain*. Oxford University Press, Oxford.

Chong, M.S. (2002). Headache syndromes presenting with facial pain and autonomic features. In eds Zakrzewska, J.Z., Harrison, S.D. *Assessment and management of orofacial pain*, pp 209–345. Elsevier, Amsterdam.

Chong, M.S. (2002). Other neurological causes of head and face pain In ed Zakrzewska, J.Z., Harrison, S.D. *Assessment and Management of Orofacial Pain*, pp 385–403, Elsevier, Amsterdam.

Drangsholt, M., Truelove, E.L., Yamuguchi, G. (2005). The case of a 52-year-old woman with chronic tooth pain unresolved by multiple traditional dental procedures: an evidence-based review of the diagnosis of trigeminal neuropathic pain. *Journal Evidence Based Dental Practice*, **5**: 1–10.

Dworkin, R.H., O'Connor, A.B., Backonja, M., Farrar, J.T., Finnerup, N.B., Jensen, T.S., Kalso, E.A., Loeser, J.D., Miaskowski, C., Nurmikko, T.J., Portenoy, R.K., Rice, A.S., Stacey, B.R., Treede, R.D., Turk, D.C., Wallace, M.S. (2007). Pharmacologic management of neuropathic pain: evidence-based recommendations. *Pain*, **132**: 237–51.

Evers, S., Afra, J., Frese, A., Goadsby, P.J., Linde, M., May, A., Sandor, P.S. (2006). EFNS guideline on the drug treatment of migraine – report of an EFNS task force. *European Journal Neurology*, **13**(6): 560–72.

Hunder, G.G., Bloch, D.A., Michel, B.A., Stevens, M.B., Arend, W.P., Calabrese, L.H., *et al.* (1990). The American College of Rheumatology Criteria for the classification of giant cell arteritis. *Arthritis Rheumatology*, **33**: 1122–8.

Loder, E., Rizzoli, P. (2008). Tension-type headache *British Medical Journal,* **336**: 88–92.

Merskey, H., Bogduk, N. (1994). *Classification of Chronic Pain. Descriptors of chronic pain syndromes and definitions of pain terms*, 2nd ed. Seattle: IASP Press.

Morillo, L.E. (2004). Migraine Headache, *BMJ Clinical Evidence*, **11**:1 696–719.

Silver, N. (2005). Headache (chronic tension-type). *BMJ Clinical Evidence*, **14**: 1610–9.

Useful websites

American Headache Society (http://www.americanheadachesociety.org/)

British Association for the Study of Headache (http://www.bash.org.uk)

Clinical Evidence (http://clinicalevidence.bmj.com)

European Federation of Neurological Societies (http://www.efns.org)

International Headache Society (http://www.i-h-s.org)

World Headache Alliance (http://www.w-h-a.org)

156

Chapter 12

Trigeminal autonomic cephalalgias

Steven Graff Radford and Suthipun Jitpimolmard

Key points

- The trigeminal autonomic cephalalgias which include cluster headache, paroxysmal hemicrania, SUNCT – short lasting neuralgiform headaches with conjunctival injection and tearing are rare causes of facial pain
- A comprehensive history and examination including baseline measure of pain and quality of life is crucial for diagnosis
- MRI for chronic unresponsive cases
- Indomethecin test to confirm presence of paroxysmal hemicrania
- Medical management: includes acute management and prophylaxis
- Psychological support important and access to written information is helpful
- Provide details of patient support group.

12.1 Chapter plan

Figure 12.1 is an outline of the main contents of this chapter.

12.2 Definition

The trigeminal autonomic cephalalgias (TACs) is a term introduced in the second edition of the International Headache Society (IHS) classification. This is a group of headache syndromes which have in common short lasting severe unilateral headache attacks and are accompanied by cranial autonomic symptoms. The term was coined to reflect excessive parasympathetic activity once triggered by trigeminal nociceptive input.

The TACs include:

- cluster headache
- paroxysmal hemicrania
- short lasting unilateral neuralgiform headache attacks with conjunctival injection and tearing (SUNCT).

Figure 12.1 Chapter plan

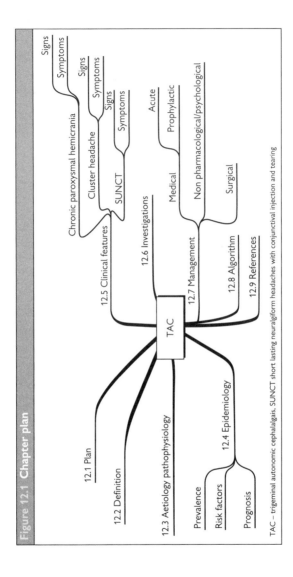

TAC – trigeminal autonomic cephalalgias, SUNCT short lasting neuralgiform headaches with conjunctival injection and tearing

12.3 Aetiology and Pathophysiology

Any pathophysiological construct for TACs must account for the two major shared clinical features characteristic of the various conditions that comprise this group: trigeminal distribution pain and ipsilateral cranial autonomic features.

The pain producing innervation of the cranium projects through branches of the trigeminal and upper cervical nerves to the trigeminocervical complex from whence nociceptive pathways project to higher centers. A reflex activation of the cranial parasympathetic outflow provides the efferent loop.

12.4 Epidemiology

12.4.1 Prevalence and Incidence

Cluster headache prevalence is less than 1% and may be autosomal dominant in about 5% of cases and start between 28–30 years. For unknown reasons men are afflicted 3–4 times more often than are women. However the opposite is found for paroxysmal hemicrania and it tends to occur in young adults and has no genetic link, its prevalence is not known, may be 2%. SUNCT is even rarer.

Night time occurrence is usual. The most common presentation that can arise is pain with autonomic features occurring multiple times per day lasting weeks to months.

12.4.2 Risk factors, risk groups

The most frequent co-existing disorder is sleep apnoea.

12.4.3 Prognosis

Remission periods are variable. Up to 10% of patients may develop chronic symptoms and after 15 years 80% of patients will still have attacks.

12.5 Clinical Features

159

These are based on the IHS criteria which have in the most part been validated by case control studies although as more studies are added some of the timing features are changing. The three conditions are compared and contrasted in Table 12.1.

Table 12.1 Diagnostic features of trigeminal autonomic cephalalgias, all are unilateral

Condition	Age onset gender	Site radiation, type	No attacks daily	Duration of attacks	Autonomic features	Precipita-ting factors	Investigation
Cluster	30 M	Peri-orbital, temple Boring, throbbing	1–8	15–180 mins	Must be present	Smoking, alcohol, altitude, REM sleep	MRI Sleep study
CPH	20 F	Peri-orbital, temple Boring	1–40	2–30 mins	Present	Neck movement	Indomethacin trial MRI
SUNCT	30 M	Orbital temporal Stabbing	1–200	10–240 seconds	Tearing, conjunctiv-al injection	Cutaneous triggers	MRI
SUNA	20 F=M	Orbital temporal Stabbing	1–30	250 seconds	May be some	None	MRI

CPH chronic paroxysmal hemicrania; SUNCT short lasting unilateral neuralgiform headache attacks with conjunctival injection and tearing, SUNA short lasting unilateral autonomic headaches, M – male, F – female

12.5.1 Chronic Paroxysmal Hemicrania
The clinical features of paroxysmal hemicrania are shown in Figure 12.2.

12.5.2 Diagnostic criteria
A At least 20 attacks fulfilling B-E
B Attacks of severe unilateral orbital, supraorbital, or temporal pain lasting 2 to 30 minutes
C Attack frequency above 5 a day for more than half of the time, although periods with lower frequency may occur
D Pain is associated with at least one of the following signs/symptoms on the pain side:
- Conjunctival injection and/or lacrimation
- Nasal congestion and/or rhinorrhea
- Ptosis and/or miosis
- Restlessness or agitation
E Headache is stopped completely by indomethacin
F Not attributed to another disorder.

If there are periods of remission with remission periods of 1 month to 3 years after a period of attacks between 2–18 weeks it is termed episodic.

12.5.3 Cluster headaches
The clinical features of cluster headache are shown in Figure 12.3.

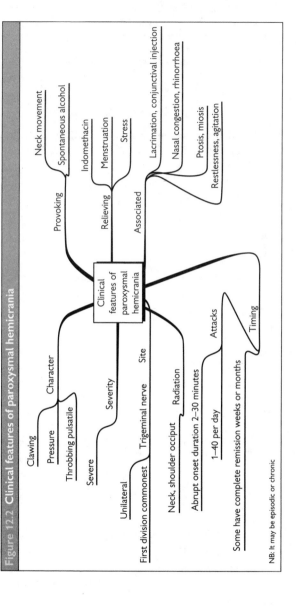

Figure 12.2 Clinical features of paroxysmal hemicrania

NB: It may be episodic or chronic

Figure 12.3 Clinical features of cluster headaches

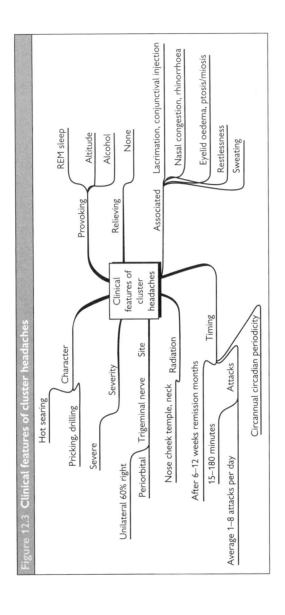

Diagnostic criteria:

A At least 5 attacks fulfilling B-D.

B Severe unilateral orbital, supraorbital and/or temporal pain lasting 30 to 180 minutes untreated for more than half of the period (or time if chronic)

C Headache is accompanied by at least one of the following signs that have to be present on the side of the pain:

- Conjunctival injection and/or lacrimation
- Nasal congestion and/or rhinorrhea
- Miosis and/or ptosis
- Restlessness or agitation

D Frequency of attacks: from 1 every other day to 5 per day for more than half of the period/or time if chronic

E Not attributed to another disorder.

The description of the pain is often very characteristic: a red hot poker pushed and twisted in or around the eye. The descriptors chosen from the McGill Pain Questionnaire are thermal and punctuate with no descriptors from the dull category. Attacks of pain build up within 5–10 minutes and reach a peak that last for up to 2 hours but 45 minutes seems the average. Classically the attacks happen within 90 minutes of the patient going to sleep and coincide with REM sleep. It tends to also occur as patients relax at the end of the day and characteristically happen at the same time and so have been termed alarm clock headaches. There is also a seasonal periodicity – around the longest and shortest days of the year. Some forms of cluster are episodic with remission periods up to five years whereas others are chronic with few remission periods.

Alcohol is a major trigger. Tearing is the most common autonomic feature. Up to half the patients will have a Horner's syndrome during the attack. In contrast to patients with trigeminal neuralgia cluster headache patients are very restless during an attack and will pace and rock. Patients may also experience migrainous symptoms such as nausea, photophobia, phonophobia and osmophobia.

12.5.4 **SUNCT Shortlasting Unilateral Neuralgiform Headache with Conjunctival Injection and Tearing**

The clinical features of SUNCT are shown in Figure 12.4.

Diagnostic criteria:

A At least 20 attacks fulfilling B-E

B Attacks of unilateral orbital, or temporal stabbing, or throbbing pain lasting from 10–120secs

C Attack frequency from 3 to 200/day

D Pain is associated with conjunctival injection and lacrimation.

E Not attributed to another disorder.

Figure 12.4 Clinical features of short lasting unilateral neuralgiform headaches with conjunctival injection and tearing

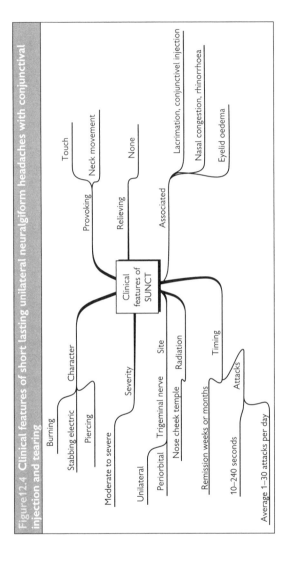

The attacks come on suddenly and there is no pain between attacks. The frequency of asymptomatic periods varies and can be as short as weeks but can be years. The autonomic symptoms are much shorter lasting then in the other conditions. It is rare for migrainous features to be present but there can be cutaneous triggers.

There is a disorder similar to SUNCT where the cranial autonomic features are other than conjunctival injection and tearing. This is called SUNA and is listed in the appendix of the International Headache Society Classification. It requires the presence of only one autonomic feature accompanying the pain. It also needs to be differentiated from first division trigeminal neuralgia.

12.6 Investigations

Imaging of the brain is not essential in episodic cluster headache where MRI's detect no more than 1 in 100 cases of lesions. However, in chronic cluster headache, an MRI is recommended because of the difficult long term management and the potential for invasive therapies. The TAC's need to be differentiated from secondary TAC producing lesions. An MRI of the brain with attention to the pituitary fossa and cavernous sinus will detect most secondary causes.

Functional imaging studies have shown activation in the hypothalamus in trigeminal autonomic cephalalgia.

12.7 Management

Summarized in Table 12.2.

12.7.1 Pharmacology

12.7.1.1 *Acute therapy for cluster headache*

- Sumatriptan 6 mg subcutaneous is the most effective acute remedy, maximum 2 doses in any 24 hour period. It is the only acute therapy that is FDA approved. It is less effective in the chronic cases. Although the other triptans may be effective, cluster's short duration may render them clinically ineffective as they take longer to absorb. Using the nasal spray preparations may also improve effects but it is not as quick acting.
- Oxygen 100% at 7 litres per minute used with a re-breath mask for 10 minutes at the onset of pain may abort attacks
- Ergotamine – best nasal aerosol
- Triptans – zolmitriptan 10 mg nasal spray
- Lidocaine as spray but not effective on its own
- Other drugs tested in RCTS but not effective have included intranasal civamide, sumatriptan oral, sodium valporate.

Other drugs that have been reported to be effective but have not been tested in RCTs include:

- Olanzapine 5–10mg orally
- There are a whole range of drugs that have been used for the acute phase which do not appear to be effective.

Table 12.2 Frequently used drugs used in trigeminal autonomic cephalalgias

Drug/therapy	Daily Dose range	Efficacy NNT very good, good, low	Side effects	Comments
Cluster headache				
Proven in RCTs and effective				
Sumatriptan	6 mg SC	NNT 2.1	Dizziness	Acute
Sumatriptan	20 mg intranasal	Good	Nil	Acute
Oxygen	7–12 L/min for 15–20 mins	Very good	Nil	More effective in younger patients, expensive
Zolmitriptan	5–10 mg oral or nasal	Good		Acute for episodic and need 10mg
Dihydroergotamine	1mg nasal spray	NNT 4.4		
Verapamil	240–960 mg	Very good	Constipation, hypotension, gastro-intestinal	Prophylaxis, monitoring ECG
Lithium	600–1200 mg	Very good	Cognitive, mood alteration, renal	Prophylaxis regular monitoring important
Commonly used but no RCT				
Lidocaine	4% intranasal	Good	Few reported side effects	Acute
Olanzapine	2.5–10 mg	Good	Drowsiness	Acute
Methylergonovine	0.2–0.8 mg	Very good	Vessel constriction Gastrointestinal irritability Uterine cramping	Used now that methysergide not available in USA
Steroid	20–80mg for three weeks	Very good	Mood change, gastrointestinal sensitivity, relapse common when doses reduced	Short term prophylaxis

Divalproic sodium/valproate	250–2000 mg	Good	Weight gain, hair loss, tremor	Prophylaxis, not available in UK
Topiramate	100–300 mg	Good	Cognitive, paresthesias, kidney stones, glaucoma, weight loss	Prophylaxis for chronic cases
Chronic Paroxysmal Hemicrania				
Commonly used and effective				
Indomethacin	25–300 mg	Very good	Gastro-intestinal discomfort Bleeding	Used in prophylaxis use H2 antagonist
Topiramate	25–200 mg	Good	As above	Used in prophylaxis
SUNCT/SUNA				
Commonly used but no RCT				
Gabapentin	300–3000 mg	Good	Sedation	
Topiramate	25–300 mg	Good	As above	
Lamotrigine	25–400 mg	Low	Rash	
RCT randomised controlled trial NNT number needed to treat				

12.7.1.2 *Prophylactic treatments for cluster headache*

As the attacks can be very frequent prophylactic treatments are used to suppress or shorten the cluster bout and must be initiated early at the start of an episode.

• Verapamil – when doses over 240mg daily are used then electrocardiographic monitoring should be done regularly

• Lithium is effective especially in chronic cases but regular monitoring is essential

• Steroids 60–100 mg for 5 days and then gradually reducing over three weeks by 10mg daily have been reported in case series

• Methylsergide was an effective drug but due to its severe side effects it has now been withdrawn .

Divalproic sodium or valproate can be effective in the short term. Open studies suggest that topiramate can be effective. Dose begins with 25 mg once a day and needs to go up to a maximum of 200 mg, according to clinical response and tolerability.

Other prophylactic drugs, many only tested in open labeled studies, have included pizotifen, nimodipine, baclofen, melatonin, gabapentin, clonodine and naratriptan.

Two drugs can be combined if treatment is not effective but the chance of side effects rises.

12.7.1.3 *Paroxysmal hemicrania*

As is described in the inclusionary criteria chronic paroxysmal hemicrania must respond to indomethacin. Initially small doses of 25 mg daily should be employed increasing daily to the minimum effective dose. Usually, indomethacin is dosed between 150 mg and 200 mg daily. A high does is needed initially and then it can be reduced. Due to the potential gastric side effects it is useful to prescribe a H2 antagonist or misoprostol. The triptans do not appear to be effective and other analgesics may be needed. Use of topiramate has been recently described in a case presentation. The dose used was 150 mg and cessation of the drug resulted in a recurrence of the pain. Alternatively verapamil and other NSAIDS can be used.

12.7.1.4 *SUNCT*

There is no one agent that has been exceptionally effective in SUNCT. Drugs used include in order of use: lamotrigine, gabapentin and topamirate. Previously used were carbamazepine and steroids.

12.7.2 **Non-Pharmacologic**

It seems logical to advise patients to avoid known trigger factors during episodes of cluster which would include:

- Alcohol
- Change in sleep habits and naps
- High altitudes including aeroplane travel.

12.7.2.1 *Nerve Blocks*

Blockade of the occipital nerve for cluster has been described recently as being effective.

12.7.2.2 *Psychological*

Psychological support for these patients has not been described but measures advocated in Chapter 5 section 5.5 may be useful for these patients. There are support groups for these patients and these are listed in Chapter 5.

12.7.3 **Surgery**

This should only be contemplated in cases with strictly unilateral headaches and all reports are case series.

Gamma Knife therapy has been used in recalcitrant patients. There is still no consensus as to the specific benefit of this therapy. The long term outcome of gamma therapy has not been established.

Gasserian ganglion rhizotomy and Gasserian ganglion gangliolysis procedures similar to those used in trigeminal neuralgia have been described and used in a few patients with SUNCT with some success.

The report of microvascular decompression (as for trigeminal neuralgia) has been described in case reports. A concern is in the differential diagnosis of SUNCT and trigeminal neuralgia. Current high resolution imaging may help provide information as to the presence of vascular loops adjacent to the trigeminal tract in the posterior cranial fossa. Specific request for this information is required as the vascular loop is not abnormal, but when present may allow the clinician to contemplate surgery. There is one case report of thalamic brain stimulation in a SUNCT patient that was beneficial.

12.8 Algorithm

Figure 12.5 is a suggested algorithm for management of the TACs based on recent guidelines. There are few RCTs due to the rarity of the disease.

Figure 12.5 **Algorithm for management of trigeminal autonomic cephalalgias**

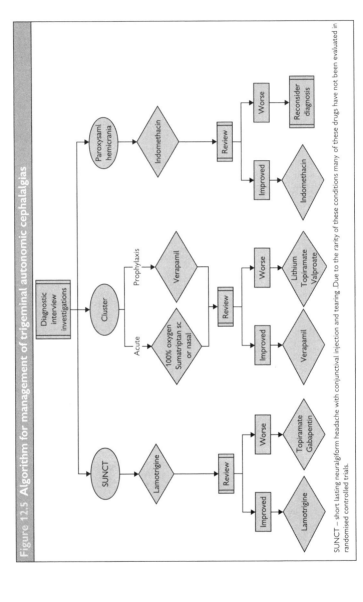

SUNCT – short lasting neuralgiform headache with conjunctival injection and tearing .Due to the rarity of these conditions many of these drugs have not been evaluated in randomised controlled trials.

Anonymous (2004). Headache Classification Subcommittee of the International Headache Society. The International Classification of Headache Disorders: 2nd edition. *Cephalalgia*, **24** (Suppl 1): 9–160 .

Bahra, A., Goadsby, P.J. (2003), Diagnosis and mismanagement of cluster headaches. *Acta Neurologica Scandinavica*, **109**: 175–9.

Chong, M.S. (2002). Headache syndromes presenting with facial pain and autonomic features . In Zakrzewska, J.M., Harrison, S.D. (eds): *Assessement and Management of Orofacial Pain*, chap 12. Amsterdam, Elsevier pp 209–45.

Manzoni, G.C. (1998). Cluster headache and lifestyle remarks on a population of 347 male patients. *Cephalalgia*, **3**: 21–30.

May, A., Leone M., Áfra, J., Linde, M., Sándor, P.S., Evers, S., Goadsby, P. J. (2006). EFNS guidelines on the treatment of cluster headache and other trigeminal-autonomic cephalalgias *European Journal of Neurology*, **13**: 1066–77.

Russell, M.B., Andersson, P.G., Thomsen, L.L., Iselius, L. (1995). Cluster headache is an autosomal dominantly inherited disorder in some families: a complex segregation analysis. *Journal Medical Genetics*, **32**: 954–6.

Sjostrand, C., Waldenlind, E., Ekbom, K. (2000). A follow up study of 60 patients after an assumed first period of cluster headache. *Cephalalgia*, **20**: 653–7.

Chapter 13

Orofacial pain disorders – linking phenotype to genotype

Christian S. Stohler

Key points

- Pain medications are consumed at disturbing rates
- Black box warnings are issued for pain medications by regulatory agencies, indicating that a fresh new science is needed
- The efficacy of most procedures and devices appears to be little different from a credible placebo
- Orofacial pain conditions are increasingly reconceptualized as complex diseases in which genes and environmental factors mediate vulnerability
- Advancing the understanding of complex diseases depends on valid phenotype-genotype linkages
- Current taxonomies appear to be too narrowly defined, leaving important phenomenological variations unscored
- Disagreements in genotype-phenotype studies have to be expected due to type I and type II errors
- To advance science, the field needs to embrace broad system's screens.

13.1 Chapter plan

Figure 13.1 is an outline of the main contents of the chapter.

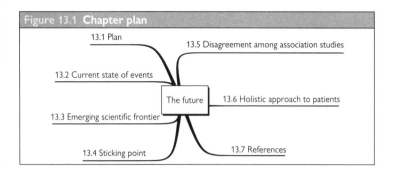

Figure 13.1 **Chapter plan**

13.1 Plan

13.5 Disagreement among association studies

13.2 Current state of events

The future

13.6 Holistic approach to patients

13.3 Emerging scientific frontier

13.4 Sticking point

13.7 References

13.2 **Current state of events**

According to the US Food and Drug Enforcement Agency (FDA), Americans are consuming pain pills at a disturbing rate. In the past year, more than 200,000 pounds of prescription codeine, morphine, oxycodone, hydrocodone and meperidine were legally dispensed, enough to give an excess of 300 milligrams to every living person in the United States. Regarding over-the-counter (OTC) painkillers, their common misuse is linked to liver failure and stomach bleeding, fatal outcomes not excluded. Through aggressive consumer advertising, blockbuster prescription pain medications may have reached select groups of people that exhibit greater susceptibility for complications than the study cohorts for which the drugs were originally approved. In light of these developments, the FDA added 'black box' warnings to all prescription and OTC pain relievers. Highly popular OTC pain killers, such as acetaminophen and non-steroidal anti-inflammatory drugs (NSAIDs), including aspirin, ibuprofen, naproxen and ketoprofen are included in the list. Similar – but not identical – rulings were released by the European Regulatory Agency.

On a broader scale, the situation surrounding pain medications is compounded by the stark realization that common procedures and devices, aimed at relieving orofacial pain and dysfunction, are overshadowed by questions regarding their efficacy and safety. This includes the many types of occlusal appliances that are widely administered by dental practitioners. Although these devices and their supporting ideas are appealing, the implied mode of action is in question as there is no difference in their effectiveness from a credible placebo.

Simple, uni-causal explanatory models of disease have dominated both the research and clinical practice of the orofacial pain conditions for much of the past century. However, the lack of response differences between treatments, targeting presumably very different mechanisms, raises concern about the validity of the theories in support of these therapies (e.g. repositioning of the articular condyle in glenoid fossa to achieve condylar concentricity; repositioning of anteriorly displaced disks to normalize the function of the condyle-disk complex; adjustments of dental occlusion to eliminate the slide from centric relation contact to centric occlusion; increasing the vertical dimension of the dental occlusion to harmonize masticatory force distribution; stabilization splints to eliminate harmful tooth contact and/or bruxism; and others). The issue that these treatments produce similar benefits – although at varying risks – no longer escapes the discussion.

While the great societal need for safe and efficacious methods to fight pain has become better understood than ever before, questions surrounding the most common ways and means to address it have become abundant. Patients' frustration is fueled by mixed messages and outright confusion. With the genomic era also came the understanding that not all subjects respond to pain the same way and many patients are wondering if their genes are to blame for their continued suffering.

Although much confusion exists about issues of safety and efficacy of current measures to deal with orofacial pain, there is renewed excitement to advance the understanding of the mechanisms that are responsible for these often disabling pain conditions. New biotechnologies make possible the measurement of the effect of disease on thousands of genes, offering unprecedented insight through a discovery process that is guided by an initial fishing expedition to zero-in on promising leads. These powerful technologies allow the exploration of new territory, invigorating the field with exciting leads.

13.3 Emerging scientific frontier

Due to recent scientific and biotechnological advances in molecular genetics and genomics, including the completion of the Human Genome Project in 2001, the possibility for exciting phenotype-genotype correlations became a reality. In fact, genetics and genomics have become the conceptual framework for advancing the science into the pathogenesis of the 12,000 diseases that affect the human race. DNA sequence variations affect the gene product and in turn, may have functional relevance in terms of either increasing or decreasing the risk of disease. There is also the broad awareness that genes are not necessarily the single most important factor in the development of disease and that environmental stimuli, including their timing (repeated, chronic, cumulative) and context within which they are presented are of importance as well. With respect to the interaction between genes and the environment, it is possible that the effect of the exposure to an environmental pathogen is conditional upon a person's genotype, or alternatively, that genes modulate the effect of environmental exposures.

Recognizing the deficiency of past centuries' uni-causal explanations of disease, there is growing endorsement for the view that the persistent orofacial pain conditions represent complex diseases in which genes, environment, and gene x environment interactions contribute to the development of disease. This modern view endorses the framework that underlines all complex diseases in which the susceptibility to disease is explained by:

1. Vulnerability genes
2. Genes that amplify an existing polygenic risk
3. Genes that exacerbate the negative effect of an environmental risk factor and/or risk-conferring behavior (Figure 13.2).

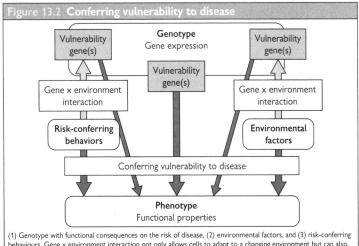

Figure 13.2 Conferring vulnerability to disease

(1) Genotype with functional consequences on the risk of disease, (2) environmental factors, and (3) risk-conferring behaviours. Gene x environment interaction not only allows cells to adapt to a changing environment but can also confer risk by transcribing genes that increase vulnerability.

In this respect, it is understood that people's predisposition to disease is conferred by combinations of genes and environmental interactions, and rarely mediated by the action of a single gene. The greater the number of genes involved, the more complicated it becomes to identify the causal sequence of events and related mechanistic treatments.

As mentioned above, today's biotechnologies open the discovery process to new levels of mechanistic insight. Low density microarrays permit rapid gene expression profiling that focus on a particular molecular pathway or host of candidate genes. High density microarray platforms allow the measurement of the expression of thousands of genes simultaneously for a given cell type, providing new clues about the underlying biology. The molecular toolbox for attributing variations in function to genes has become so powerful that the obstacles to advancing the science, given the use of sound molecular protocols and standards to define the genotype, have become much less of an issue than the availability of valid protocols to characterize the clinical phenotype.

The establishment of meaningful genotype-phenotype correlations is always a challenge as it depends on the sensitivity and specificity of measures by which the phenotype is assessed and classified, and the validity of the molecular processes that lead to the identification of the genotype. Differential gene expressions between cells of normally common genetic background, e.g. cancerous/non-cancerous, where individual cells are morphologically identified and harvested using single cell caption devices, provide information of change in gene function as a result of disease. However, for complex human diseases with syndromal presentation, such as the persistent orofacial pain conditions, current understanding does not allow linking of symptoms and clinical signs to a particular cell type of interest. Consequently, the discovery process into their causation is a challenge.

Although progress has been made with respect to the development, refinement and standardization of measures to classify clinic cases involving orofacial pain, the construct within which current disease taxonomies force case assignments appears to be not as comprehensive as it should be to produce meaningful genotype-phenotype correlations.

Based upon the body of the literature of the past 15 years, strong reliance on anatomical structures and topographical domains do not appear to be useful as those characteristics (e.g. trigeminal tract involvement V1, V2, V3, or muscle, joint, disk) seem to have little predictive value for the course of the disease, e.g. trigeminal neuropathy or TMJ disease, treated or not. Diagnostic taxonomies need to capture and be founded on those distinguishing features that are consequential for stratifying cases into subsets for which mechanistic differences in the underlying pathogenesis have to be assumed.

Regrettably, scientific inquiries are largely driven by disciplinary entitlements and territorial stakeouts. In this respect, a tight anatomical focus, imposed by disciplinary constraints, limits the diagnostic case assignment to criteria that are observable in the discipline's primary field of interest, a matter of great concern to temporomandibular diseases and disorders (TMJDs). While the domain concept, which localizes a disease-related abnormality to a particular topographical area, calls for the detailed case workup in the region of interest, symptoms and signs outside the topographical domain applicable to dentistry/orofacial pain are customarily not acknowledged. If they are, it is of little significance to case assignment and/or case management. This is most apparent in those tertiary patients for whom the burden of disease is shaped by troubling comorbidities and which happen to constitute the case majority as only 15% of patients seeking care for reasons of facial pain in a specialty clinic have their symptomatology limited to the face domain.

The fact that the literature defines the phenotype in narrow terms, limiting the description to a set of traits within a topographical domain that is 'owned' by a particular discipline has a direct bearing on gene discovery. For example, symptom generators outside the territory claimed by the respective discipline may influence the patient's complaints and possibly the clinical features within the region of interest. However, the present state of science views these comorbid traits as statistical and not biological entities because little is known how these phenomena are mechanistically linked. When asked about their present pain intensity, not referencing any particular body site, women with widespread pain, seeking treatment for facial pain, reported generic present pain intensity scores of which the most intense pain site in the body explained 82%, the average intensity across all pain sites 62%, and the most intense pain site in the face 61% of the variation (Figure 13.3).

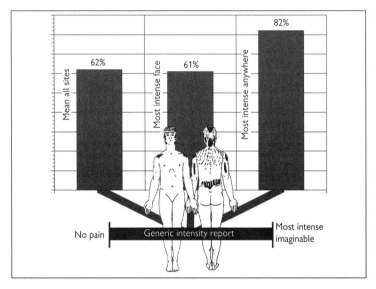

Figure 13.3 Variation in generic pain intensity scores of women seeking care for facial pain in a specialty clinic is explained by the most intense pain anywhere in the body (82%) to a greater degree than averages of pain intensities across pain sites (62%), or even the most intense pain in the face (61%). See text.

The significance of imposed 'turf' boundaries on diagnosis and treatment is illustrated in Figure 13.4 showing the neck involvement of cases, diagnosed as RDC/TMD Type I conditions.

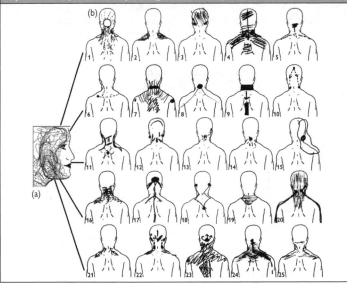

Figure 13.4 Individual drawings of the neck pain distribution of patients diagnosed with RDC/TMD Type I (N = 25). The disciplinary focus represents a powerful reporting bias

Correctly or not, face involvement has always been viewed as the primary or characteristic manifestation. Any neck participation is treated as secondary and conceptualized as complication or spread of disease to adjacent tissue. In addition, many of the late stage systemic complaints, often shaping the burden of disease and impacting on the patient's overall well-being in a major way, are not unique to the persistent orofacial pain conditions and occur with many other chronic ailments. The fact that those past decades of caring for complex orofacial pain patients has left much to be desired when it comes to serving those with the greatest disease burden, calls for fresh new thinking.

However, while insufficient acknowledgment of the broader body pain topography is of concern, the limited scope of characterizing the persistent orofacial pain phenotype constitutes a much broader issue than just a matter of bodily pain distribution. As sensory, motor, autonomic, affective and cognitive systems are activated to varying degrees from patient-to-patient, driving many of the comorbid complaints, the limitation of a set of anatomically-based, non-functional criteria that define the phenotype and criteria for case assignment must be recognized.

While the utility of the most advanced classification system for TMJDs, the RDC/TMD taxonomy is suited for the phenotypic delineation in epidemiologic field studies, the research instrument was never intended to be applied to the other side of the clinical spectrum at which late genes and their gene products are in effect in conditions that are confounded by comorbid phenomena involving sensory, motor, autonomic, affective and cognitive systems (Figure 13.5).

In these complex cases of persistent pain with concomitant additional ailments and ancillary features, the sole dependence on the RDC/TMD diagnoses does not seem to be appropriate for phenotype-genotype correlations as the assigned diagnosis may provide little information about the complex biology in effect.

13.5 **Disagreement among association studies**

Genotype-phenotype association studies are prone to establish statistically significant results that may or may not be replicated in subsequent work due to both type I errors, declaring evidence in favor of an association when in truth there is none, or type II errors, the failure to declare a significant biological effect when one truly exists.

Allelic association means that the occurrence of an allele with the disease phenotype is either significantly increased or decreased in statistical terms from random incidence. Reasons of non-confirmation include:

• The play of chance
• Deficient sample size
• Allelic and/or phenotypic heterogeneity of the study sample
• Misclassification of the genotype and/or phenotype.

Phenotypic heterogeneity refers to the fact that the clinical presentation expresses itself differently in different subjects while genetic heterogeneity is present when different genes cause clinically indistinguishable presentations.

Regarding the phenotype, linkages may not be confirmed in subsequent work if the threshold of disease is different between studies as the odds ratio that defines either protection or risk for a given gene variant depends on the

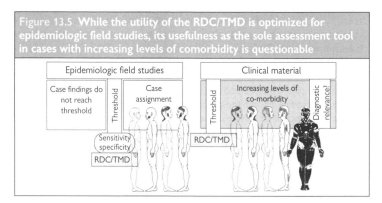

Figure 13.5 While the utility of the RDC/TMD is optimized for epidemiologic field studies, its usefulness as the sole assessment tool in cases with increasing levels of comorbidity is questionable

operational definition of the phenotype. As noted above, significant differences between study samples may exist with respect to disease severity and comorbidity, even within a given diagnostic RDC/TMD subset (e.g., type I, II, III), which may be the reason for non-replication. Another reason may be due to differences in the racial/ethnic makeup of the study samples as different groups may exhibit both different allele frequencies as well as culturally-mediated reporting biases.

Regarding the genotype, problems with the validation of protocols and/or reagents (e.g., oligonucleotide probes based on poor sequence data), or differences between microarray platforms, such as the validity of cross platform comparisons of gene expression data, may also be responsible for disagreements among primary studies. Furthermore, the effect of the gene variant may be conditional on the exposure to an environmental pathogen and/or risk-conferring behavior that may be expressed at a higher level in one study samples and not the other.

Once a sufficient body of literature is available to examine whether an allelic influence is genuine or not, the strength of the statistical evidence across studies, including the estimation of the allelic effect size is appraised employing meta-analytic methodologies, appropriately combining primary studies to arrive at a summary conclusion. Although a few genes and their gene products have been linked to conditions of orofacial pain, the number of primary studies, often reporting disagreement as one might expect, remains insufficient to allow the execution of a formal meta-analysis at this time.

13.6 Give your patient a complete physical examination

As the persistent orofacial pain conditions are increasingly being viewed by scientists, professionals and patients as complex diseases comparable to diabetes, Alzheimer's disease or cardiovascular disease, cracking the puzzle of genetic and environmental factors that impact on the causal sequence of events has become the goal for research for the next two decades. What is the proportion of risk that is attributed to a specific allele, and what are the chances for the disease to be expressed if the allele is present?

In order for the 21st century molecular tools to become meaningful for genotype-phenotype correlations, the point has been reached where we need to give our patient a complete physical examination, without bias with respect to scope of practice or the provider's favorite choice of treatment as systemic abnormality may produce artifacts of disease-specific measures. No different from phenotyping a genetically engineered mouse, we need broad system's screens and a range of functional assays to characterize the unique individual characteristics present in the state of disease for the purpose of elucidating the role of genes. What other disease, as devastating as the persistent orofacial pain states can be, gets no or little of a routine physical examination, including the assessment of body weight, body temperature, pulse, heartbeat, vision, hearing, neurological reflexes, neuromuscular measures, mood, eating, sleeping and others? The clinical assessment paradigm needs to be refreshed and to be aligned with the tools that have the power to break the disease code, little by little.

Acknowledgements

This work was supported by NIH/NIDCR RO1 DE15396 (CSS).

13.7 References

Dworkin, S.F., LeResche, L. (1992). Research diagnostic criteria for temporomandibular disorders: review, criteria, examinations and specifications, critique. *Journal of Craniomandibular Disorders*, **6**: 301–55.

Kreiner, M., Betancor, E., Clark, G.T., Kreiner, M., Betancor, E., Clark, G.T. (2001). Occlusal stabilization appliances. Evidence of their efficacy. *Journal of American Dental Association*, **132**: 770–7.

Turp, J.C., Kowalski, C.J., O'Leary, N., Stohler, C.S. (1998). Pain maps from facial pain patients indicate a broad pain geography. *Journal. Dental Research*, **77**: 1465–72.

Turp, J.C., Kowalski, C.J., Stohler, C.S. (2000). Generic pain intensity scores are affected by painful comorbidity. *Journal Orofacial Pain*, **14**: 47–51.

Appendix

A plan of the Appendix is shown in Figure 14.1.

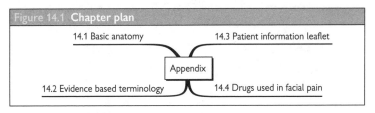

Figure 14.1 Chapter plan

14.1 Basic anatomy   14.3 Patient information leaflet

Appendix

14.2 Evidence based terminology   14.4 Drugs used in facial pain

14.1 Anatomy

See Figure 14.2. Cranial nerves shown diagrammatically on the ventral surface of the brain and the major entry points of the cranial nerves.

14.1.1 The trigeminal nerve, fifth cranial nerve

This is primarily a sensory nerve made up of three major divisions as shown in Figure 14.3.

The top smallest branch, known as the ophthalmic division, often annotated as V1 or VA, provides sensation to the forehead, eyes and the bridge of the nose. The middle branch, which is called the maxillary division, shortened to V2 or VB, supplies sensation to the inside of the mouth in the region of the upper jaw, upper teeth, lips, cheeks and palate, sinuses and also on the skin of the cheek and the nose. The third division, called the mandibular division, also referred to as V3 or VC, supplies sensation inside the mouth to the lower jaw, lower teeth, lower lip, the front of the tongue and outside of the skin and part of the ear. It does not supply sensation to the skin at the angle of the jaw.

The nerve then passes forward to the Meckel's cave where there is a large crescent-shaped ganglion, the Gasserian or semilunar ganglion. Meckel's cave can be identified on the skull by an impression near the apex of the petrous part of the temporal bone. It then enters the brain in the posterior fossa at the pons as shown in Figure 14.2.

The motor division of the trigeminal nerve which emerges from the skull through the foramen ovale, supplies temporalis, the masseter, the medial pterygoid and the lateral pterygoid as well as anterior belly of digastric and mylohyoid. It also supplies motor sensation to the tensor veli palatini and tensor tympani which open and close the Eustachian tube which equalizes pressure between the middle and inner ear.

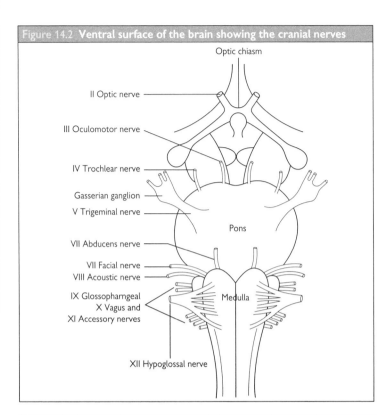

Figure 14.2 **Ventral surface of the brain showing the cranial nerves**

Optic chiasm

II Optic nerve

III Oculomotor nerve

IV Trochlear nerve

Gasserian ganglion
V Trigeminal nerve

Pons

VII Abducens nerve

VII Facial nerve
VIII Acoustic nerve

IX Glossopharngeal
X Vagus and
XI Accessory nerves

Medulla

XII Hypoglossal nerve

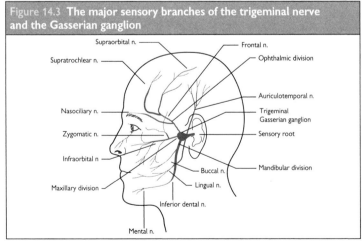

Figure 14.3 **The major sensory branches of the trigeminal nerve and the Gasserian ganglion**

Supraorbital n.

Supratrochlear n.

Nasociliary n.

Zygomatic n.

Infraorbital n

Maxillary division

Frontal n.

Ophthalmic division

Auriculotemporal n.

Trigeminal
Gasserian ganglion

Sensory root

Mandibular division

Buccal n.

Lingual n.

Inferior dental n.

Mental n.

14.1.2 **Facial nerve – seventh cranial nerve**

This nerve supplies the muscles of facial expression and emerges from the brainstem between the pons and the medulla. The 7th nerve also supplies taste to the anterior two thirds of the tongue. The submandibular gland and sublingual glands are supplied via chorda tympani with parasympathetic fibres from the seventh nerve.

14.1.3 **Structure of nerve fibres**

Figure 14.4 shows the structure of different nerve fibres.

185

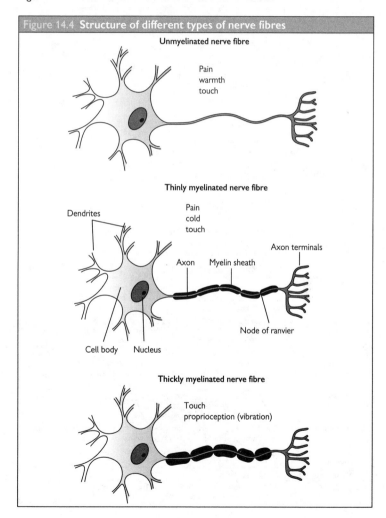

Figure 14.4 Structure of different types of nerve fibres

14.2 **Evidence based terminology**

Table 14.1 lists the major terms used in evidence based medicine.

Table 14.1 Glossary of terms used in evidence based medicine based on Evidence Based Dentistry Journal and Cochrane Collaboration

Term	Definition
Case control study	Compares a group with the disease/condition to another group from the same population who do not have the condition
Case series	A report based on a series of patients with condition with no control group, there may be independently derived objective measures
Cohort study	A clearly identified group is followed up for a period of time, it can be retrospective or prospective
Cross over trial	A trial in which all participants will receive the treatment but in random order
Efficacy	Extent to which a treatment improves outcome for patients under ideal circumstances
Intention to treat	Results are analysed according to intended treatment to which a patient was allocated in a randomised controlled trial rather than to the actual treatment received
Levels of evidence	Hierarchy of evidence of trials which determines the rigour of the study: systematic review, RCT, case controlled trial, case series
Meta-analysis	A statistical method of summarising several studies into a single estimate
Number needed to treat NNT	Number of patients needed to treat for a specific intervention to see occurrence of a specific outcome e.g. pain relief. The lower the number the more effective the intervention
Number needed to harm NNH	Number of patients needed to treat for a specific intervention before an adverse event occurs. The lower the number the more likelihood that a patient will have a side effect
Odds	Ratio of probability of an event occurring to that of it not occurring
Odds ratio OR	Measure of clinical effectiveness or adverse events. If OR = 1 then effect of intervention no different from control, if OR is > or < then the effects of the intervention are more (or less) than those of the control intervention
Probability value P	Determination of whether the results are just due to chance. If p value is <0.05 then the result is not a chance finding and the result is statistically significant
Randomised controlled trial RCT	A trial in which subjects are randomly assigned to an intervention group or to a control group in which everyone is blinded to the assignment. They are then followed up to determine if there are any differences between the groups
Relative risk or risk ratio RR	Risk of experiencing a particular result. A RR >1 means there is an increased risk while >1 suggests decreased risk. The higher the number the more likely is the particular result
Responders in pain trials	Responders to treatment are defined as those who achieved a 50% reduction in pain which may not be complete pain relief
Risk difference or absolute risk	This is the difference in size of risk between two groups
Recommendations	These are based on levels of evidence that have been determined
Systematic review	A review in which all the evidence has been systematically gathered, appraised and then summarised using pre-determined criteria

14.3 Example of patient information leaflet

The leaflets are produced on A4 sheets that can be folded into three so as to make it easy to slip into a pocket or bag. Below is an example of leaflet for burning mouth syndrome.

14.3.1 What is Burning Mouth Syndrome (BMS)?

This condition is characterized by a burning pain or hot sensation, which can be localized to the lips or tongue or more widespread in the mouth. The burning can be continuous or intermittent. It can be accompanied by other symptoms like dryness or an unpleasant taste, or feelings of numbness. The burning can increase with talking, eating hot or spicy foods, and in times of stress. It can be lessened by some foods or drink, sleep, or rest and distraction. It is a very real symptom.

In the research literature Burning Mouth Syndrome is sometimes referred to by other names such as glossodynia, glossopyrosis, or stomodynia oral dysaesthesia.

14.3.2 Who gets it?

Depending on which study you read, between 0.75% and 15% of the population are affected. Typically we see 2 or 3 patients each week in this clinic. It is more common in women than men. The women most commonly affected are those around the menopause.

14.3.3 What else causes burning in the mouth?

Burning mouth can be caused by diseases or by a deficiency (shortage) of vitamins or minerals. It is not caused by cancer.

When we first see you in the clinic we will carry out a detailed examination of your mouth to exclude any disease. We may take a mouth swab if we suspect that you may have a candidal (fungal) infection. We will then take some blood and carry out tests for levels of iron, vitamin B_{12}, folic acid, and glucose. If we find any abnormality, treating the underlying disease may improve your symptoms. When the results of all these investigations are normal then a diagnosis of Burning Mouth Syndrome (BMS) is made.

14.3.4 What causes BMS?

The cause of BMS is poorly understood. Recent studies suggest that in sufferers, changes occur in the way the tongue transmits sensations of warm, cold and taste to the brain. This leads to the pain, discomfort, or burning. It is called a neuropathic pain as it is caused by malfunctioning of nerves. The effect of these symptoms may be to alter the production of hormones in the blood which can lead to altered sleep habits, fatigue and depression. Burning is NOT a symptom of mouth cancer.

14.3.5 **What are the effects of living with BMS?**

Living with ongoing physical symptoms is difficult. Those people who seem to do best develop ways of trying to make sure they carry on with the things they enjoy in life as much as possible, despite the symptoms. This sometimes means actively challenging thoughts such as 'having a meal is not the same as it used to be'. While this may have truth in it, it is still possible to take enjoyment from activities, but we may have to re-focus on how enjoyable it is to share the food with friends, or appreciate smells etc.

Some people find that the symptoms of BMS cause them to feel low or stop doing things they used to. If this is the case for you, you can seek further help from our specialised team of health psychologists. Health psychologists can support people in being able to have a good quality of life, despite these types of difficulties.

14.3.6 **What treatments are available?**

The most important part of the treatment is to accept that this is a long term condition and may take a number of years to disappear. It is very important to develop some coping strategies. Relaxation, yoga and meditation will all help. Make sure you set aside time to do pleasurable activities and reward yourself if you have coped well with the day. These types of measures are as important as any medication we currently have available.

As with all chronic pain, low dose antidepressants can be helpful if taken over a year or two. Your specialist or GP could prescribe them. Other anticonvulsive drugs such as gabapentin and clonazepam have been used, but only a few patients will benefit from their use.

In trials it has also been suggested that alphalipoic acid, a dietary additive, may be useful for BMS. The dose suggested is 200 mg 3 times daily for a month and then one daily. It can be bought in health food shops.

Burning is often worse when accompanied with dryness. Use plain water or sugar free chewing gum to help keep your mouth moist.

It is useful to keep a diary to see how your symptoms respond to the treatments you use.

Further information

Ask your specialist for further information or look in the Cochrane collaboration for consumer summary of treatments that have been used. See http://www.cochrane.org/reviews/en/ab002779.html

Version 1, January 2008

Review date, January 2010

14.4 **Drugs**

Table 14.2 lists some of the drugs used in management of facial pain. This is not exhaustive and lists some of the trade names of the generic drugs mentioned in this book. Before prescribing any drug please check in your national formulary.

Generic name	Trade name/s used US/UK	Class of drug
Table 14.2 Some of the major drugs used in the management of facial pain		
Generic name	Trade name/s used US/UK	Class of drug
Amitryptyline	Elavil, Tripafen	Antidepressant
Baclofen	Lioresal	Antispasmodic
Capsaicin	Axsain, Dolorac, Capzasin-P, Zacin	Analgesic, topical
Carbamazepine	Tegretol, Tegretol retard, Teril retard, Timonil retard, Atretol, Carbatrol, Epitol	AED
Clonazepam	Rivotril, klonopin	Tranquilizer
Codeine phosphate	Codeine	Opioid
Divalproex	Depakote	AED
Dosulepin	Prothiaden	Antidepressant
Fentanyl	Actiq, Duragesic	Opioid
Fluoxetine	Prozac	Antidepressant
Gabapentin	Neurontin	AED
Imipramine	Norfranil, tofranil	Antidepressant
Indometacin (Indomethacin)	Indocid	Analgesic
Lamotrigine	Lamictal	AED
Leviteracetam	Keppra	AED
Lidocaine	Xylocaine, EMLA	Analgesic
Lithium carbonate	Camcolit, Liskonum, Priadel	Antimanic
Morphine	Oramorph, Seredol, Morcap, Morphagesic, MST Continus, MXL, Zomorph	Opioid
Nortriptyline	Allegron, Pamelor	Antidepressant
Oxcarbazepine	Trileptal	AED
Oxycodone	OxyNorm, OxyContin	Opioid
Phenytoin	Dilantin, Epanutin	AED
Pimozide	Orap	Antipsychotic
Sumatriptan	Imigran	Triptan
Tiagabine	Gabitril	AED
Tizanidine	Zanaflex	Muscle relaxant
Topiramte	Topamax	AED
Valproic acid	Depakene, Depakote, Epilim, Convulex	AED
Venlafaxine	Effexor	Antidepressant
Verapamil	Cordilox, Securon	Anti-angina
Zolmitriptan	Zomig	Triptan
Zonisamide	Zonergan	AED
AED anti-epileptic		

Index

A

abscess, dental 72
acetaminophen 174
acupuncture 19, 115, 116,
    127t, 140, 152, 154, 189
AED (anti-epileptic drug) 189
almotriptan 151t
alphalipoic acid 89, 90t
alprazolam 57
alveolar osteitis 73
amisulpride 90
amitriptyline 58, 89, 102t, 140,
    189
amoxycillin 78
analgesics 57, 140
anatomy
    cranial nerves 183, 184f
    facial nerve 185
    Gasserian ganglion 184f
    nerve fibre structure 185
    trigeminal nerve 183, 184f
anti-epileptics 59, 140,
    152, 189
anti-inflammatories 75, 152
    see also NSAIDs
antibiotics 72, 73, 78
anticonvulsants 59, 101
antidepressants 52, 58, 89,
    115, 115t, 140
antipsychotics 90, 189
anxiety 38, 51, 85, 88,
    98, 113
anxiolytics 90
AO see atypical odontalgia
aspirin 76t , 154, 174
assessment,
    social/environmental 21
atypical facial pain see chronic
    idiopathic facial pain
atypical odontalgia (AO)
    aetiology/pathophysiology
        95
    clinical features 96, 97
    definitions of 93, 95
    epidemiology 95–96
    investigations 96, 98
    management 98
    see also chronic
        (persistent?) idiopathic
        facial pain; traumatic
        induced neuralgia
atypical trigeminal
    neuralgia 122

B

baclofen 125, 126, 167, 189
Beck Depression
    Inventory 40
benzodiazepines 57–58, 115t
benzydamine chlorhydrate
    90
beta blockers 152
blood investigations
    results, interpretation of 29t
BMS see burning mouth
    syndrome
bone scintigraphy 33
botulinum toxin 152
Brief Pain Inventory 41
**burning mouth syndrome
    (BMS)** 7, 50
    aetiology/pathophysiology
        85
    blood investigations 27
    clinical features 86–88
    coexisting disorders 27
    definition of 83
    drug levels 27
    epidemiology
        frequency 7
        prognosis 86
        risk factors 86
    haematological
        abnormalities 27
    investigations
        drug history 88
        haemotological/
            biochemical 88
        immunological tests 88
        microbiological 88
        potential causes, exclusion
            of 88, 89t
        sensory tests 88
    management
        algorithm 91f
        pharmacological
            therapies 89–90
        psychological
            interventions 91
        patient information
            leaflet 91, 187–88
        renal/liver functions 27

C

calcium channel ligands 59,
    140, 142, 152

capsaicin cream 57, 89, 101,
    140, 189
carbamazepine 125, 126, 140,
    168, 189
caries, dental 6, 34, 71–72
Cartesian 'amputation'
    approach 71
catastrophizing 41, 64
cavernous sinus
    thrombosis 154
CBCT (cone beam computed
    tomography) 98
celecoxib 56
chlodiazepoxide 90
**chronic idiopathic orofacial
    pain**
    frequency 6, 7–8
    misdiagnosis of 51
    radiological investigation
        32, 55
    special characteristics
        of 55
chronic pain model 62–63
**chronic paroxysmal
    hemicrania (CPH)** 160t
    clinical features 161
    definition of 157
    diagnostic criteria 160
    management 167t, 168
civamide 165
classification systems
    dental/oral mucosal pain
        disorders 47, 48
    musculoskeletal pain
        disorders 47, 48–49
    neurovascular orofacial
        pain disorders 47,
        49–51
clomipramine 89
clonazepam 57, 89, 90t, 125,
    126, 189
clonodine 167
cluster headaches
    clinical features 160t, 162,
        163
    definition of 157
    non-pharmacologic
        treatment 168
    pharmacological treatment
        acute 165–66
        frequently use drugs
            166–67t
        prophylactic 167–68
codeine 174, 189